EXECU-CIZE

by Perry Howard

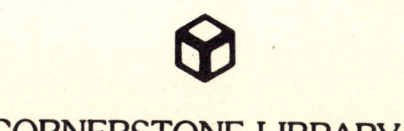

CORNERSTONE LIBRARY

Copyright © 1979 by Cornerstone Library, Inc.

All rights reserved, including the right of reproduction
in whole or in part, in any form

Published by Cornerstone Library
A Simon & Schuster Subsidiary of
Gulf & Western Corporation
Simon & Schuster Building
1230 Avenue of the Americas
New York, New York 10020

The trademark of Cornerstone Library, Inc. consists of the words
"Cornerstone Library" and the portrayal of a cube and is registered
in the United States Patent Office

Manufactured in the United States of America

ISBN 346-12389-5

CONTENTS

Introduction: Exercise! Who's Got Time To Exercise? 1
1 The Executive Myth 3
2 The Return on Your Investment 8
3 What's So Great About Muscles? 14
4 What Is Fitness? 25
5 Learn the Exercises 37
6 Tips and Hints for Execucizing 42
7 The Core Exercises 56
8 Good Morning, Good Evening 85
9 Grace Under Pressure 88
10 When the Telephone Rings 108
11 Execucizes for Special Occasions 124
12 Sample Programs 136
13 The Company Cafeteria 149
14 How Long Will All This Take? 158
15 Execucize as a Group Activity 160

INTRODUCTION

EXERCISE! WHO'S GOT TIME TO EXERCISE?

You do, that's who! With this program, anyway. It is this very fact that makes Execucize unique. It was designed with you—the busy executive in mind. I know that every successful businessman and woman really needs twenty-five hours in every day and eight days in every week. That is why a sound program of regular exercise is one of the first things dropped from an overcrowded calendar. In the attempt to get everything done that must be, the typical executive tends to view physical activity as a luxury that is too expensive in terms of time, or worse, as frivolous. Something that is simply not necessary.

Well, exercise is neither. It is not a luxury. Far from

EXECU-CIZE

it. Rather it is a necessity. And it is not frivolous. What necessity of life ever is? Exercise, on a sound, regular basis, is as essential to your continued well-being as are air and water. And I have yet to meet the executive, however busy, who is prepared to forego air and water. So why give the axe to physical fitness?

That is a question which brings us back to the ever-present stumbling block of the modern executive—time. Where does the time come from? It doesn't. You already have the time available to you. Every time you walk into your office, you can exercise. Every time you sit down at your desk or at a conference table, you can exercise. Every time you pick up a telephone to make or take a call, you can exercise. Every time you dictate a letter, you can exercise.

This program is the wish fulfillment of the modern business community. It allows all of us who earn our livings by sitting at a desk to do two things at the same time and yet to do them both well. That is where the time you need comes from. You combine two activities into one. You get yourself back into shape, and stay that way, while you are pursuing your career. If you've got the desk, you've got the time!

CHAPTER 1

THE EXECUTIVE MYTH

Quick! In three words or less, name the most over-worked, underexercised segment of the American population. Come on, now. Who are these men and women? Can't think of an answer? Do you give up? The answer is: The Modern American Executive! That's right. You! If you work in an office, sit behind a desk, and spend most of your time thinking, planning, writing reports, and making decisions, you are very likely to be overworked and underexercised. Yes, you, a member of one of the more prestigious segments of our society.

In a way it is ironic that an admired, if not actually envied, group of people could be in such a poor state, especially since most Americans are trying to achieve just the opposite—less working time so as to have more time left over for leisure activites. What happened to the

EXECU-CIZE

American executive? Actually, nothing much. Business people have always worked hard leaving themselves little, if any time, for exercise. Unfortunately, though, a myth began to grow up around what executive life was like. I used to believe that myth as much as the next person. Then I started on my career and found out differently.

When I began college, I decided on business partly because I had a knack for it, partly because I felt that it was the field that offered the most opportunity, and partly because I liked the life I thought I was going to lead. Executives, to my way of thinking, had it made. They lived a soft, comfortable life.

The way I saw it, Joe Executive lived in a nice apartment, drove a late-model car, wore stylish clothes, and gave "fun" parties. He also strolled into the office between 9:15 and 10:45 and strolled out again any time after 4:00 so as to avoid the rush-hour crowds. Between Monday and Friday, he had a two-hour lunch at some fashionable restaurant. On weekends, he went sailing, fishing, golfing, or something like that. But above all, he always looked good. Not too heavy, not too thin. All that weekend exercise kept him that way.

It did not work out that way, or at least not exactly. I did get myself a nice apartment, a late model car, and a few stylish suits. As for the rest of it—wellll. I have to admit there wasn't too much trouble with the rush-hour crowds because I was usually way ahead of them or behind them. None of this strolling in between 9:15 and 10:45 and then out again shortly after 4:00. Ordinarily I'd get to the office between 8:15 and 8:30 so I could get

THE EXECUTIVE MYTH

some work done without interruptions. If I left at six o'clock, I considered that I had left the office early. As for the famous three-martini lunch in a fashionable restaurant, I considered myself lucky if I could sneak away to the company cafeteria for a somewhat dry and tasteless sandwich washed down with a cup of weak coffee.

As for those weekends devoted to leisure-time activities—ha,ha! I had lots of things to keep me occupied, and they had nothing to do with the "high life." The work I took home with me, for example. Or waiting for those frantic phone calls from my boss. The ones that went something like this, "The XYZ report absolutely has to be done by Monday morning, and I just found some errors in the figures. You'd better meet me at the office in an hour so we can get this thing straightened out." On those really good weekends, when there wasn't more work waiting for my attention, I would just catch up on my sleep. My tennis racket and golf clubs gathered dust in the closet. Every now and again, I'd look at them and promise myself that the coming weekend I would find time to use them. I never found the time for the exercise. Within a few years, this lack of exercise began to show.

I was no longer in the great shape I had once been in. I was getting soft around the middle, and around a few other places, too. And I was gaining weight. Not a lot of extra poundage, but enough to be annoying. Most of the people with whom I worked had the same problem. Their physical shape reflected the lack of exercise. What is more, they all admitted, when pressed, that they never thought it would happen to them. But I think you know what I'm talking about. You are probably living just this way right now. After all, you are reading this book. You may, however, be a bit confused about the whole thing. You may be wondering, "What happened? How did it happen? What did I do wrong?"

Among my friends who found themselves in the same state I was in, there was an underlying sense of guilt about their poor physical condition. They believed that they were somehow at fault. They could not, of course, pinpoint just where they made their mistake, but they were convinced that they had made one. Subconsciously, they were still subscribing to The Executive Myth that they had it "made" once they took up their post behind a desk, and that they had all the time in the world to do what they wanted. You may be silently accusing yourself for letting your physical condition deteriorate. My advice to you is: Stop it. You are not really at fault because there is a basic fact of life, one from which there is no escape. Men and women who choose business careers work hard. They have, as I mentioned before, always done so. They will probably continue to do so. The popular myth is very nice and very pleasant, but it has absolutely no connection with reality.

Anyone who wants to make a success of a business career has to work hard. Another popular form of reasoning among my friends goes something like this, "I'm lazy. That's why I don't exercise. What other reason is there?" Laziness does not even enter the picture. Successful business people are not lazy. Rather, they are just the opposite. They are unusually hard working. They

THE EXECUTIVE MYTH

routinely put their careers before their personal wants, and even, needs.

One of these needs happens to be exercise. Only through regular, practical exercise can you stay in top shape. But you are not necessarily at fault because you do not get enough exercise. It is part of the price you have to pay if you are to have a successful career. Or it was until now!

Fortunately, though, the situation is changing. It is no longer necessary to neglect exercise. It can be fitted in very easily with your current lifestyle. No longer is it necessary for you to trade off the need to work hard by cutting down on your physical activities. You can combine the two, and this is what this book is all about.

CHAPTER 2

THE RETURN ON YOUR INVESTMENT

As an executive, I really cannot ask you, another executive, to accept my proposition without giving you some idea of why you should make this investment in physical fitness and what you stand to gain from it. You have been trained to look very closely at proposed plans before committing yourself. You want to know the ins and outs and the ups and downs before you give your approval. Blind faith is not the stuff of which a solid business career is built. It is not, either, the stuff of which good health and fitness are made. For many executives, bulging belly becomes something they accept and live with. They may not like it, but they cannot see the advantage in correcting it. They can, however, see quite clearly the disadvantages. A physical fitness program means, they believe, a large investment of TIME. They do not have the time on hand. As I

THE RETURN ON YOUR INVESTMENT

explained, the time IS available, but there is still the question of what sort of a return will come from this investment.

A few pages back, I mentioned that business is a demanding career. To truly make your mark, you need every ounce of energy you can squeeze out of your body and brain. The better the shape of your body, the greater the amount of energy you will have at your disposal. And when you have vast reserves of stamina from which to draw, your thinking is more likely to be clear and logical and your planning more effective and original. All of these positive features add up to a successful career. No one, then, can deny the need for energy and physical stamina. But where does it come from, especially when you are out of shape? Vitamin pills? A tablespoon of tonic? Doubtful, very doubtful, indeed. There is no vitamin tablet or bottled tonic, whether a patent or prescription compound, that can ever substitute for good old fashioned physical fitness.

And here I speak from personal experience. I tried that route myself. For about a year, I faithfully swallowed a widely advertised vitamin tablet and choked down an equally well-known tonic. The stuff certainly didn't do me any harm, but then it didn't do me much good either. Nothing happened—I ended as I started, a tired, flabby businessman. And if I hadn't accepted the fact that solid physical fitness achieved through a program of regular exercise was the only way to increase my stamina, I would probably still be chugging along sagging and dragging in all the wrong places.

But along with increased stamina, genuine physical

EXECU-CIZE

fitness also pays another valuable dividend in terms of your continued good health. To complement the reserves of energy, the up and coming modern business executive also needs health, health, and more health. A heavy cold, a bout with the flu, a run-in with the season's most popular virus can throw your work schedule off by as much as a month. My last bronchiole infection, as my doctor called it, cost me five days home from the office. My staff did a terrific job of covering for me, but still, when I got back to work there was a mound of paper waiting to greet me. Over two weeks went by before I finally caught up with it all. And only then by working harder than I would have if I had been on schedule. In the long run, that so-called bronchiole infection cost me more than five days flat on my back.

These colds, lung infections, whatever you want to call them, can also mean more than time lost at the office. The can also mean some of the glitter lost from your image as a member of the business community. Quite recently an acquaintance of mine was expounding on this very point. Hank had a cold, but because he also had an appointment with a very important client, he came into the office, gathered up his material, and dashed off to his meeting. As Hank later told me, "The old so and so practically threw me out of his office. There wasn't one grain of sympathy from him as I sat there blowing my nose and wiping my eyes. You know what he said? 'I really wish you hadn't come in here in this condition. I neither want nor need your germs.' Can you imagine the nerve of that guy?"

Yes, frankly, I can. Who, after all, wants to talk

THE RETURN ON YOUR INVESTMENT

business with someone whose mind is on reaching for tissues and not on the matter at hand? Like it or not, Hank made a very poor impression that day. And that is something that would not have happened if he had not had that cold. While I cannot guarantee that you will never be sick again if you get back into shape, I can say that you will probably be less likely to get sick. After all, statistics show that those who are in top-notch physical condition are less likely to fall ill. Good health is proving to be less of a luxury and more of a necessity in the business world, isn't it?

Which brings us around to my next point. Speaking subjectively, I think business is one of the most satisfying careers available to today's bright men and women. And the longer the career lasts, the greater the satisfaction that becomes available. The key word here is "longer." Poor physical fitness does nothing to lengthen your business career and, in extreme cases, can even shorten it. This fact was brought home to me rather brutally one afternoon when my secretary rushed into my office and announced in a stunned voice, "Mr. Hennning just died. He had a heart attack in the airport waiting room. Isn't that awful?" Yes, it was awful, particularly since Jack Henning was only forty-seven years old with a good twenty years of promising future before him. Jack was also terribly out of shape and had been so for about ten years. He did not take care of himself and that neglect played a large part in cutting off his career.

But that is what poor physical condition can do, it can cost you the very thing you value and want to make the most of. But even if you manage to hang on by

11

EXECU-CIZE

dragging your sagging body around with you, you are not really helping your career. Having a wide-ranging mind can get you a super promotion; having a wide-ranging mid-section can get you stuck in the corporate basement.

Business corporations, like almost everyone else, go out of their way to project a positive image. They want to look their best for the customers, for the clients, for the competition. Public relations is an important aspect of modern business practice. As a consequence, business corporations also want their employees, particularly their executive employees, to project a positive image. There is very little room for Sammy Sag and Fanny Flab in this scheme of looking great for the public.

And the ironic thing is that there are dozens of stories around that support my position. At one convention I attended, I bumped into a fellow whom I knew slightly, and he started to fill me in on the promotional problems he was having back at the "shop." "There's one guy I'd really love to bring along, but everytime I suggest him, the vice-president puts his foot down," he remarked.

"What's wrong with the guy?" I asked. "Nothing that can't be corrected. My company has an image of being dynamic and strong. They are always looking for sharp people who fit in with this image. This man I'm talking about doesn't fit the corporate image. He looks as though he hasn't the strength to pick up a tube of toothpaste. Until he gets back into shape, he's not going anywhere within the company. Too bad, because he's really got the ability to hack it." Think back for a moment on your own career. Have you perhaps been passed

THE RETURN ON YOUR INVESTMENT

over for a promotion you wanted, and, what's more, deserved? Many of us, I suspect, have experienced such a disappointment. But think a bit more, could the reason have been because you did not fit easily into the image the company wished to project? Is the poor, unattractive condition of your body holding you back?

But what other dividends can be had from a sound, regular program of physical fitness? A very human dividend. A sense of accomplishment, of achievement. There is a great deal of pleasure to be had when you can say, honestly, "I've done something really well!" Getting yourself back into shape and then maintaining that condition can allow you to feel that pride, that satisfaction. This pride, in turn, leads to something else that is equally as valuable. A sense of self-confidence. Knowing that you look well and feel well can do wonders for your ego. It can provide that extra "shot in the arm" that so many of us lack.

All in all, I firmly believe that some very important and necessary dividends can be had from a program of regular physical fitness. While I cannot guarantee that you will receive all of these dividends because no solid, blue-chip investment ever makes such guarantees, I do know that if you don't try for physical fitness, you will never achieve any of the benefits. The only way to derive all the good things that come from sound physical conditioning is by putting yourself back into sound physical condition. It is as simple as that! This is one program where you have absolutely nothing to lose except your tight white collar. And while doing that, there is a good chance that you will gain a great deal more—more than you ever realized that you would!

CHAPTER 3

WHAT'S SO GREAT ABOUT MUSCLES?

Quite a bit, actually, because without them you could not function as a human being, much less as an executive. Simply turning the pages of this book requires muscle power. Signing a contract, buzzing your secretary, giving instructions to your staff, all of these actions require you to use your muscles. Unfortunately, we use some muscles more than others. And this fact, in turn, contributes to poor physical fitness. As an example of what I am saying, let me mention the muscles in our fingers. Very few people have poor muscle tone in this area because their fingers are in almost constant use. Think about that for a moment. How many times have you tapped your fingers on your desk impatiently or toyed with a pencil or doodled on a pad? The dozens of "nervous" habits that we all have,

WHAT'S SO GREAT ABOUT MUSCLES?

however annoying to others, serve to keep the muscles of our fingers in great shape.

Yet despite the importance of our muscles, they are generally neglected. Even during a physical examination, you come away with the feeling that you have only one muscle worth worrying about—your heart. Most company physicals these days include an electrocardiogram as a matter of course. And this is as it should be; your heart is *the* most important muscle that you have; your heart is the only muscle that is *essential* to your continued life. Naturally, there must be constant monitoring for heart disease—as well as for high levels of cholesterol and blood pressure. Both, by the way, are terms that are bandied about quite a lot these days, but they are rarely defined and explained.

Cholesterol is nothing more than a waxy substance that is found throughout the body, particularly in the brain, nervous tissue, and in the adrenal glands. The liver produces some of the cholesterol; the rest we acquire from certain foods such as animal fats, dairy products, and eggs. Lately, cholesterol has come to have a negative connotation. Label a food as being low in cholesterol or better yet, as having none, and the public rushes out to buy the item. A complete absence of cholesterol, however, is as dangerous as too much because this substance plays an important role in the repair of ruptured membranes and in the formation of sex hormones and bile acids.

The levels of *normal* blood cholesterol can actually vary greatly among individuals. To determine what is normal, a physician has to consider several factors such

EXECU-CIZE

as age, sex, race, hormone production, climate, and occupation. Generally, though, the level of blood cholesterol is believed to be dependent on the amount produced by the body itself. An over-abundance of cholesterol can be caused by stress situations. Tension sets the adrenalin glands to work; if the adrenalin is not used, the surplus forms cholesterol. What we eat, of course, plays an important part, too. Yet the actual cholesterol content of our diet may be less significant than the fat content. Simply switching to polyunsaturated fatty acids (of the type found in most vegetable oils) seems to accomplish very little. There should also be a corresponding reduction in saturated (animal) fats if the level of blood cholesterol is to be lowered.

If cholesterol does serve a useful purpose, why are there high levels of such great concern? Because there seems to be a connection between the substance and atherosclerosis. Where high levels of cholesterol are present, heart disease is more common. The lower the level, the less likelihood of heart trouble. The precise reason for this is not yet known. What is known, however, is that when atherosclerosis is found, so are large deposits of cholesterol on the arterial walls.

High levels of cholesterol can also lead to high blood pressure as can overeating, obesity, smoking, *lack of exercise,* and *stress and anxiety.* And it is a well-known fact that the higher the blood pressure, the greater the risk of atherosclerosis. Just why is not yet precisely known either. Some experts think that it is because the pressure of the blood forces the cholesterol to adhere to the arterial walls. Others feel that the high

WHAT'S SO GREAT ABOUT MUSCLES?

blood pressure is a symptom and not a cause. All agree, however, that *aging* does *not* cause it. But whatever causes high blood pressure matters less than what it does.

Having high blood pressure definitely means that excessive and unnecessary strain is being exerted on the heart muscle, the coronary arteries, and the whole arterial system. The heart has to pump with greater force. If this situation is maintained over a long period of time, the heart muscle will enlarge. In men between the ages of thirty and sixty, a systolic blood pressure over 150 doubles the likelihood of a heart attack and quadruples the likelihood of a stroke.

High blood pressure itself is nothing more than the resistance of the arteries to the efforts of the heart to pump. When the heart pumps less and/or if the arteries are dilated, low blood pressure results. When the heart pumps more and/or if the arteries are constricted, high blood pressure results. It is as simple as that.

We all experience temporary high blood pressure on occasion. Excitement, stress, apprehension, anger, fear can all cause the systolic blood pressure to go up. (Exercise, too, can raise the output of the heart temporarily, but this is *not* a serious thing unless there is an *existing* and *unknown* heart disorder.) Actually, the body can, and does, withstand an occasional rise in blood pressure quite well. The trouble comes when the condition becomes *frequent* and *sustained*. And usually hypertension does become frequent and sustained in the early thirties. Although it can show up at any age, the early thirties seem to be danger time probably because it

EXECU-CIZE

is at this time of life that our careers really get moving. Aside from staying calm, blood pressure can be kept at normal levels with *exercise,* weight control, reduced salt intake when necessary.

That is why, during a physical examination, so much attention is given to your heart. As for your other muscles, they are generally ignored, because, well, who cares? You should. Your muscles play a tremendous role in your over-all health and well-being. Muscles are not only important and vital in themselves, they also exert great influence on your metabolism and on your emotional states. Use of your muscles serves to keep your heart and circulatory systems in good shape and your general energy level high.

The life of an executive, however, invites muscle neglect. The work itself is sedentary. Sitting at a desk is the hallmark of the executive. And, too, the modern office comes equipped with all sorts of gadgets and machines which are meant to save time and *energy.* What is more, there is no sign that this trend is being reversed.

Conserving energy is just great, but it is hard on the muscles. I'll give you an example. Until a few years ago, I used to have a hand-cranked pencil sharpener on my desk. It was installed to save me time. Instead of calling for my secretary each time I needed my pencils sharpened, I would just reach over and turn the handle a few times. Don't misunderstand me, I don't claim this was great exercise or that I kept my arms in top-notch condition by using it. but it was a fairly common motion for me and certainly did not do any harm. During a

WHAT'S SO GREAT ABOUT MUSCLES?

redecorating binge at my company, the little hand-turned pencil sharpener was removed and replaced by an electric one. Now even the motion of turning the handle is gone. Fewer muscles are now required to sharpen my pencils. That is an example of how office life invites poor muscle tone. There are hundreds of other examples that could be listed. What happens is that our muscles lose their strength and elasticity. The process itself is barely noticeable. Then one day, it is necessary to climb a flight of stairs. A relatively simple procedure turns out to be a major undertaking. The whole process of slipping into poor physical condition is complete. And it never should have happened.

Very few of us are born in poor physical condition. To achieve it, like anything else, we have to work at it by neglecting our muscles. A healthy, normal baby gets all the necessary exercise automatically. The baby lies in a crib and kicks its feet and waves its arms. These seemingly senseless motions are in actuality building up muscle strength. Nature has programed the child for exercise. The toddler and the school child also get their share of exercise by playing. The popular childhood games like playing ball, jumping rope, riding a bike, climbing trees are sources of the natural exercise of childhood. With this kind of a background, how can anyone get out of shape? We grow older and assume adult responsibilities.

Poor physical fitness usually begins to develop during the late teen years with those who are NOT athletic. The automobile replaces the bicycle or two feet as the most popular mode of transportation. For people

EXECU-CIZE

who are not athletic, this can be a physical disaster where muscles are concerned, because this is often the only form of exercise these people ever receive. For the more athletic types, the muscles begin to lose shape once they start working. Time then becomes a problem. Where there were once evenings and weekends to participate in a favorite sport, these leisure hours are now given over to a career. The fellow who was once the star of his college football team counts himself lucky if he can catch the doings of his favorite team on television of a Sunday afternoon. Getting into pads and a helmet to kick around the old pigskin is out of the question. The rising young executive who never missed a chance to play tennis, whether on an indoor or outdoor court, can just about find time to have a favorite racket restrung. The once devoted golf player is overjoyed when an associate suggests discussing business on the links. But even in those cases, the exercise is not all that impressive. There is something called a golf cart that has become *de rigeur*. The chance to exercise while walking the course is lost. A budding college track star has a chance to recapture the by-gone days only when he is late for his train and has to dash a half a block so he won't miss it.

Some people are, sad to say, naturally lazy when it comes to their physical condition. They hate to move anywhere for any reason. These are the people who really sit up and take notice when they hear the words, "labor saving device!" Any gadget that is supposed to save them a physical motion can come along, and these people cannot wait to buy it. To be fair, the desire for labor-saving devices can be rooted in a desire to make

WHAT'S SO GREAT ABOUT MUSCLES?

more time which can then be devoted to business. I work with a fellow who is waiting most anxiously for an electric pen to be invented so that he can put the time and energy required to sign his name to "better use." Ironically, these people, the ones who neglect their muscles, are also the first ones to wonder, and very loudly, too, why they are out of shape. "With all the moving around I do," they tend to wail. "Why I'm never still." By their standards, they are not, but to them any motion, no matter how slight, is a great effort.

For the most part, though, a low level of physical fitness is the result of a lack of knowledge. Very few of us really know anything about our bodies. Oh, we know the basic parts, to be sure. Two arms, two legs. We realize that there is a set of bones that can be broken. We also know about the more important parts like the heart. And we know, too, that there are troublesome things like gall bladders that often have to be removed surgically. We are bombarded with information that too much alcohol can destroy a good liver and that smoking can ruin a perfectly good set of lungs, not to mention the heart. But we do not really know much about our muscles. They are not readily visible like arms and legs are. They do not become ulcerated like a stomach or develop stones like a gall bladder. They stay rather quiet until that day comes along when the escalator or elevator breaks down and the owner of the muscles has to climb up a long flight of stairs or, worse yet, several flights of stairs. The leg muscles exposed to this unaccustomed use begin to hurt. Nothing very serious, certainly. But enough of an ache to remind the owner that there are muscles in his body. As I

EXECU-CIZE

wrote earlier, a simple procedure becomes a major undertaking. There might be a few passing thoughts like, "I'm really out of shape. Maybe I should do something about it." If the owner of the muscles is fortunate, an exercise program will be introduced. Most people, though, forget about the problem. And that is a very easy thing to do because even the sorest of muscles will quiet down in a day or two.

The hard fact of the matter is that muscles need care and exercise. The sad fact is that very few of us know this. The more you use a muscle, the healthier that muscle will be. They were designed to be used, not to be retired while you are still in your prime. Many people have literally forgotten that they have muscles. We also live in a society where muscles do not get the respect that they deserve. How many times have you heard the expression, "muscle head," in reference to someone who is not overly bright? Or something like, "all muscle and no brain." Or so and so "muscled his way in" in reference to someone who displayed pushy behavior. It is expressions such as these which help us to develop a mind-set that comes to believe that there is something negative about muslces.

And it is only human nature to overlook those things which are not held in very high regard. There is also the problem that we simply take our muscles for granted. They are there, they do what they are supposed to do, and that is the end of the matter. They do not need care or attention. Not so. If they are neglected (which is what an absence of exercise is, plain neglect),

WHAT'S SO GREAT ABOUT MUSCLES?

they fall down on the job they are supposed to do. They do not function as they should when you need them.

Fortunately, it is never too late to counteract neglect of your muscles. You can have two years of neglect to your credit or twenty-two. It does not matter. If you begin, keep up with, and maintain a good, solid program of exercise, your muscles can be brought back into nearly top-notice shape.

There is another factor that contributes to poor physical fitness. It, like some of the other factors, is also overlooked and by the very people who should know better. Here I am referring to the experts, to those who made careers for themselves telling others how and why they should not let themselves go. As you know, this is not the only shape-up program available to you or anyone else for that matter. A quick glance along the shelves of your favorite bookstore will tell you that. You may have even tried a few of these programs. And chances are that you gave them up after a week or two. Therein lies the problem.

You gave them up after a week or two. Why? Probably the program itself was boring. The typical exercise program involves a certain number of motions. They are repeated day after day in the same order. Furthermore, anyone following the program is expected to drop everything else they may have to do and spend anywhere from thirty minutes to an hour on the program. Is it any wonder that someone would find this boring? Most people who find these programs boring do so because they are. And if they are not boring, the

EXECU-CIZE

program calls for special equipment, special clothing, special rooms in which to do the motions. None of these requirements are really practical, especially for today's busy executive. All of this is rather unfortunate, because if anyone does need a good solid program of physical fitness, it is the average, overworked, underexercised executive.

Any activity that requires you to do the same thing for a long stretch of time, such as thirty or sixty minutes, is bound to get on your nerves after a while. Execucize, on the other hand, is broken up and spread out over the course of your working day. You can do the actions whenever you want. Some people do them all in the morning, others in the afternoon, some just spread them out between the hours of nine and five. The plan is for your schedule entirely. But now I think it's time to stop talking about what exercise is, why muscles are important, and how fitness pays off. Now it's time to explain the various motions that form Execucize.

CHAPTER 4

WHAT IS FITNESS?

In terms of the broadest possible meaning, your level of physical fitness is determined by your ability to deal with your environment and the pressures it puts on you—both mentally and physically. In the more commonplace sense of the expression, your level of physical fitness is determined by the ability of your body to endure. What is more, fitness is often used interchangeably with health. The two words, however, do not mean the same thing. Your favorite athlete may be in superb physical condition and still be sick. Maybe he's laid up with a heavy cold. By the same token, someone who appears to be "the picture of health" in the sense of being without a disease that a doctor can spot, may be in terrible physical shape. The greater the endurance, however, the less likelihood of illness, whether major or minor, so in some degree health is related to fitness.

In the past, high levels of fitness could be maintained quite easily through work—plain, hard physical

EXECU-CIZE

labor, and through what is termed transport effort—getting yourself from place to place by walking, riding a bicycle, rowing a boat. If you could do the work and get yourself around, you were fit. Today, very few of us, and most certainly not the modern executive, can depend on work and transport efforts to keep us in good shape. Therefore, a program of planned and regular exercise is important. It becomes our one reliable source of physical fitness.

Actual physical fitness has four basic parts: (1) General Work Capacity, (2) Muscular Strength, (3) Muscular Endurance, and (4) Joint Flexibility.

General Work Capacity is measured in terms of your body's ability to supply itself with the oxygen and energy it needs to keep going during general physical activity. Because high levels of General Work Capacity depend on the efficiency of your cardio-vascular and respiratory systems, it is usually referred to as "circulo-respiratory fitness" or CR fitness. CR fitness is necessary for those activities which call upon a good proportion of your body's muscles over an extended period of time. For example, fast walking, running, jogging, swimming, bicycling. Your limit of CR endurance is reached when your breathing becomes labored and your heart pounds. The actual state of your muscles does not really enter into it.

Muscular Strength is measured in terms of the maximum force a particular group of muscles can apply in one action. This force is made up of two types. There is isometric strength, which is muscular force applied against a fixed resistance. In other words, there is no physical motion involved. Isotonic strength, on the other

WHAT IS FITNESS?

hand, involves motion not only from your muscles, but also from a joint or set of joints. Your ability to lift objects is an example. The greater the amount of weight you can lift, the higher your level of isotonic strength. Indian wrestling is an activity that calls for both types of strength. Both parties try to keep their arms motionless; both parties are also exerting force against an immovable object (an arm). Isotonic strength, however, is required to force an arm down to the table. While people with high levels of isometric strength usually display high levels of isotonic strength, this is not always the case. It is possible to have one type without the other.

The third component of fitness, Muscular Endurance, is measured by the ability of a particular muscle or group of muscles to continue functioning over a period of time. The longer the period of time, the higher the level of strength. As with Muscular Strength, there is also both isometric and isotonic endurance.

Isometric endurance is determined by your ability to maintain force as long as possible against a fixed resistance or to maintain yourself in a fixed position. For instance, if you were Indian-wrestling, the longer you could keep your arm up while, at the same time, applying force against your opponent, the higher your level of isometric endurance. Isotonic endurance, on the other hand, is measured in terms of your ability to repeat a particular muscular action. For example, the more push-ups you can do, the higher your level of muscular endurance. You reach your level of both isometric and isotonic endurance when your muscles simply will not respond anymore.

The last aspect of fitness, flexibility, concerns your

EXECU-CIZE

joints, i.e., elbows, knees, and the range of normal motions they will perform easily. Usually when joints are not as flexible as they might be, it is because the muscles surrounding the joint (or joints) are not as strong as they might be.

Interestingly, your levels of muscular strength and endurance and flexibility can vary from one part of your body to another. You can exhibit high levels of these components, for instance, in your legs and not in your arms. Conversely, by developing one area of your body, say your abdominal area, you will not automatically develop the other areas. But in the course of developing one area, you will raise your levels of strength, endurance, and flexibility. In other words, when you improve your muscular strength, you automatically improve your muscular endurance and joint flexibility (assuming that there is a joint in that area). Does this seem far-fetched to you? It should not because if you are right handed, you will almost certainly have greater strength, endurance, and flexibility in your right arm. This is because your right arm gets considerably more use than your left. Your level of CR fitness is, on the other hand, an independent component. You do not automatically improve your muscular strength and endurance and joint flexibility when you raise your CR level. The opposite also holds true.

Another interesting point about fitness, the higher your various levels, the longer your body can tolerate lesser challenges. Let us say that the greatest weight you can lift easily is eighty pounds. You would have an easier time lifting a forty pound weight than someone who is able to lift easily a maximum of fifty pounds.

WHAT IS FITNESS?

The actual physical capabilities of your body, however, are determined not only by your fitness, which is very important, but also by your motor abilities such as coordination, balance, agility, reaction time, speed, movement time (the speed at which you can move a part of your body), and power (your ability to perform a sudden, explosive movement).

Overall physical fitness also contributes to your efficiency in the sense that the more fit your body is the more efficiently it works. As you know, efficiency is determined by how much work will be produced from a given amount of energy. Your efficiency will vary from day to day and even from hour to hour. It all depends on how near you are to your limits. All systems, however, including yours, are more or less inefficient. When the full output range is considered, all give less than 100% return. The average human body is between 16 and 27% efficient. This compares badly with a great many machines. With regular exercise, however, the body's efficiency can be raised to as high as 56%. Very few machines can match that level.

Now that we have discussed the actual components of fitness and how they are measured, we can talk about the things which affect fitness. There are three things which do so to a greater or lesser degree.

Age is one. Each prime stage of life offers an advantage. The ability for speed usually reaches its peak during young adulthood, strength in the late twenties, and endurance during middle-age. Because most of us are not as fit as we might be, these abilities can be improved at almost any age. Even if you are forty-five right now, you can improve your rate of speed because

EXECU-CIZE

you are not as quick as you might be. You would, though, be unable to achieve the speed of a twenty-year-old.

The second thing that affects fitness is sex. Constitutionally, woman have the potential for a higher level of fitness than do men. Under normal circumstances, they are able to tolerate wider shifts in temperature; they also tend to live longer. Men, on the other hand, tend to be more specific in their fitness in that they have a greater potential for strength and speed.

And the third thing is what is called somatotype—the shape of your body. People who are tall and lean and people who are short and broad do not have the ability to achieve the same level of fitness. Both groups, though, can reach high levels—based on the potential for their particular body type.

What all this boils down to, of course, is that even if we were all at the top level of physical ability, we would all demonstrate different rates of speed, flexibility, muscular strength and endurance, etc.

As several factors *affect* physical fitness, several factors also *determine* your fitness. The first of these is your state of health. You simply cannot become or remain fit if your body is in poor health. Another is nutrition. A healthy diet is essential if you are to attain and maintain fitness and health. The third is your weight. If you are above the desirable weight for your body type, your body is constantly working under the burden of an extra load. If, however, you are too far below your ideal weight, your tissues will not have the ability to function at the highest possible level of efficiency. The fourth is

WHAT IS FITNESS?

sleep. Adequate rest is as necessary to your body—as well as to your mind—as is food and air. And the last is, of course, physical activity. When your body is denied activity, it shows signs of atrophy. This is why someone who is confined to a wheel chair will gradually lose the strength in his legs even if the reason for such confinement has nothing to do with these limbs.

But atrophy, or something like it, can occur without physical confinement. For a mechanical device, use produces wear and deterioration. For the human being, the opposite is true. While the changes that occur during strenuous activity are extraordinary, it is chiefly because of disuse that the body deteriorates. Once full physical growth has been obtained, there can be no further physical improvement without increased physical demand. This fact holds true not only for muscular strength and cardio-vascular and respiratory response, but also for motor abilities such as co-ordination and reaction time. Furthermore, an absence of physical activity not only fails to develop latent capacity, but it also results in a general deterioration throughout the body. The effects on your muscular system are the most noticeable. This is because you have 639 muscles in your body, and they account for approximately forty-five percent of your body weight. When you let your muscles go slack, you develop a feeling of overall physical weakness and tiredness, a weak and sagging abdomen, back pains because the muscles are not strong enough to do their work, and a weak heart. Of these four, two of them—weak and sagging abdomen and weak heart—are most likely to lead to further problems. Let your abdominal

EXECU-CIZE

muscles go slack, and you are inviting digestive trouble. A weak heart means a slow flow of blood throughout your entire system. That, in turn, leads to blocked arteries and capillaries.

In other words, when you are inactive, you have a reduced vitality, a lowered resistance to infection. You may also display certain mental attitudes in your lack of enthusiasm and concentration. You may also exhibit signs of irritability, nervousness, and insomnia. Physical inactivity also means that you increase the amount you eat which leads to weight gain and all its negative consequences. And when you are finally faced with physical activity of some sort, your heart is unable to increase its stroke volume. The result is a pounding heart because it is trying to keep up with the increased demand by beating faster.

When you take up regular physical activities, your body reacts in a positive way. Your motor skills improve. You are able to move more gracefully and efficiently as well as more quickly. Your reactions have more power. Flexibility also improves, although no one, as yet, understands the process by which this occurs. What is known is that improved flexibility reduces the chances of the joints being injured and of muscular stress. Of course, the reduced chance of muscular stress also has a great deal to do with the improved state of your muscles.

Activity allows them to (1) increase in size because the individual muscle fibers become larger, (2) increase in strength because of the larger muscle fibers which, in turn, prompt larger muscles, (3) increase in hardness probably because there is a tighter contraction and

WHAT IS FITNESS?

muscle tissue replaces fat, and (4) increase in endurance which is thought to result from increased capillarization and improved nervous organization.

Your heart, like your other muscles, also gains from suitable exercise. Its strength, co-ordination, and endurance improve. Because more blood is pumped per stroke, the rate of your heartbeat can be lower. In a normal adult who is at rest, the heart rate is 70 per minute, although 80 or even 90, is not unusual. A program of exercise can lower the rate to 60, or even 55 beats a minute. Furthermore, you achieve a greater number of capillaries and therefore, your blood supply improves. This means that your body cells are able to use more oxygen and nutrients. And, too, these extra capillaries allow the heart to recover more quickly from an attack.

The chances of thrombosis and varicose veins are reduced because the walls of the veins are more flexible, thus allowing the blood to return more quickly from the extremeties—your arms and legs; and because the blood does not clot as much. This more rapid flow of blood also keeps arterial deposits in check and the levels of cholesterol and fats low. Most probably because the energy needed for exercise is fueled by fats—the body draws upon its reserves.

All in all, when you take part in suitable exercise, you can reduce the likelihood of developing cardiovascular disorders; and, if they do occur, you can increase your chances of recovery. To prove this, all you have to do is check the statistics for the rates of coronary heart disease and death in active vs. sedentary occupations. So important is heart exercise that it is often recommended for those who are recovering from some form of heart disease.

Exercise can also improve and strengthen your respiratory system. Your general air intake increases in both vital capacity which is the amount that you can breathe in at one time and ventilation which is the amount you can inhale over a given period of time. The alveoli of your lungs also display a greater efficiency during the gas exchange process. There is also an increase in the number of red blood cells which improves the efficiency of gas transport.

These advantages are rather well-known, but there are other advantages that are less so. Physical activity allows you to develop better posture. Strong, firm muscles are, of course, required for good posture.

There is also an improvement in your nervous system. You are less tense and nervous because exercise allows you to work them off. And, too, your tolerance for pressure increases. You are also more alert mentally in that your concentration is better, your interpretation is too. As a result, you make decisions more quickly because you are better able to judge and respond.

Another benefit that accrues is a greater resistance to infection and injury. And should you get sick or injure yourself, you will most likely recover in less time than you would require if you were not fit. Regular exercise also plays a part in weight control because it allows you to use up excess calories and stimulates your body to waste more calories in thermogenesis (the formation of body heat).

WHAT IS FITNESS?

Furthermore, your level of energy is raised. There are four reasons for this (1) your metabolic rate is lowered so your energy reserves are not wasted, (2) your respiratory, cardio-vascular, and digestive systems operate more efficiently. This means that during some exertion, oxygen and nutrients are more quickly available to your cells. Your recovery from the exertion is also faster, too, (3) your muscles can function with a reduced supply of oxygen, if necessary, for longer periods, and (4) any form of exertion is less likely to exceed your actual capabilities. To put it bluntly, you are able to put more effort into your work for longer periods without feeling tired.

Regular exercise also has a positive effect on your life expectancy. Statistics for each age group prove this. Those who are active physically live longer than those who are not. There is no getting away from it. The more physically active you are, the better you will feel, look, and perform.

Having explained what fitness is and having assured you that exercise, or physical activity, can help you achieve fitness, I think it is only fair to define exercise because it can, and often does, mean different things to different people. For many people exercise is any motion that is hard work and that produces a sweat. Their reasoning goes something like this: "The hard work makes me sweat, and all the perspiration means I'm burning off calories." Exercise can be "hard work" in the sense that jogging and swimming are. Such efforts may even cause you to sweat, but just because you are a bit soggy does not mean you are burning off calories. For

EXECU-CIZE

other people, exercise is any activity that requires special clothing or equipment. To them tennis is a wonderful physical activity because they have to wear shorts or a brief dress and tote a racket. Climbing up a flight of stairs is not exercise to them. Certainly a sport like tennis will contribute to fitness, but so will climbing a flight of stairs. Exercise has nothing to do with the clothes you wear or the equipment you need.

Nor does exercise have to be some group activity under the direction of a leader calling out "One, two, one, two." Going back to an activity I mentioned before, climbing a flight of stairs. That can be exercise—good exercise—especially if you look for chances to climb rather than avoiding them. What is more, if you gradually increase the speed with which you climb, you gain greater benefits. Walking will do the same thing—if you gradually increase not only your distance, but also your speed.

Exercise then, is any action that causes your muscles to work harder, to move in an unaccustomed way, and to exert themselves. There are several types of physical activity. Execucize makes use of three of them (1) isometric which requires you to use one body muscle against another or against a fixed object such as a table or a desk, (2) muscular endurance exercises which are meant to increase muscle size through a repetitive "pumping" action, and (3) flexibility exercises which are made up of rotating and stretching actions that involve the arms, legs, and waist.

Sounds simple, doesn't it? It should because exercise—the source of good physical fitness and health—is simple. And this book proves it.

CHAPTER 5

LEARN THE EXERCISES

When I was putting this program together, I deliberately selected actions that were simple—not only simple to do, but also simple to learn. In my experience, the average executive already has more than enough to learn, remember, and do that is complicated, if not plain difficult. But however simple these motions are, they do have to be learned first. Before you start the program in your office, go through the exercises in your home, or if you belong to one, your club or gym. Learn them fully so that you can do them without thinking.

This is an important part of the Execucize Program, being able to do the exercises without thinking about them. And, too, these exercises are not simply for your body for the sake of motions. Each action involves a particular group or set of muscles. As you practice to learn the exercises, you will also have a chance to find out which of your muscles are called into play and how. When you are aware of how your muscles react, you will be able to see the value of each exercise. Furthermore,

EXECU-CIZE

you will also be able to decide which action or actions are most suited to *your* needs.

There is, too, a way to learn the exercises.

1.

Read the instructions for each action at least twice so that you are certain of how it must be done to achieve the maximum benefit.

2.

Practice the motion before a mirror. This will permit you to see just what you are doing and to know whether or not you are doing it correctly.

LEARN THE EXERCISES

3.

While you are learning the motions, move your body slowly and deliberately. Many people make the mistake of moving too quickly. This is not a wise thing to do for a number of reasons. Their bodies are out of shape and therefore unaccustomed to sudden and extreme strain. A pulled or even a torn muscle is most likely to be the result of moving too quickly too soon. Furthermore, by moving too fast, even when working before a mirror, they cannot "watch" how the exercise is done. In short, they cannot study the swing and sway of their bodies; they cannot judge whether or not they are doing the exercise properly. And even if they manage to avoid these drawbacks, they are likely to tire themselves out before they actually start the program. This unnecessary exhaustion usually leads to a sense of discouragement with the whole idea of getting back into sound physical condition.

EXECU-CIZE

4.

Try each motion at least three times to be sure you are doing it properly. (I cannot emphasize this enough, because poor or sloppy execution of a motion achieves next to nothing.) And, too, this allows you to decide just which execucizes you find most enjoyable. Very frankly, you probably will not like doing every action described in this book. You are not expected to. Some of these execucizes will appeal to you more than others will. Do not let this worry you. There are certain to be at least a dozen actions that you like. Concentrate on doing these. If you should find that all the motions described appeal to you—well and good. These practice sessions in your own home will also allow you an opportunity to identify those areas of your body which need special consideration. Not everyone is built the same way and not everyone's muscles go slack in the same way either. Some people are in need of a general physical fitness program; others have to concern themselves with two or three areas; and others, just one particular area. While you are learning the execucizes, you can also use the opportunity to take a good, long look at yourself in the mirror and decide how you stand when it comes to physical fitness. If you decide that only one particular area, say your abdominal area, is out of

LEARN THE EXERCISES

shape, then you can concentrate on learning the stomach execucizes first.

Another thing, take your time when learning the actions. Do not expect to have all the execucizes down pat in thirty minutes. The order in which you study and practice is up to you. Many people find the easiest way to pick them up is to do one section at a time. Others prefer to take *one* execucize at a time from *each* section and learn those. How you choose to learn is up to you. There is no hurry. It is far better if you take a week or ten days and really learn the exercises than if you hurry through in a day or two and then start the program without being fully prepared. This practice time also serves to introduce your body to regular exercise on a gradual basis. Those unused muscles can be "broken in." A lack of complete preparation is another good way to end up with sore and aching muscles, not to mention a sense of discouragement. And now for one final point.

I am often asked whether it is a good idea to learn these execucizes to music. I say "no" because you will not have an opportunity to do them at the office to music. I feel it is far better if you establish your own rhythm. Enough. I think you have all the information you need. As I mentioned at the beginning of this chapter, the execucizes are not only easy to learn, but also easy to do. Now I'll prove it.

CHAPTER 6

TIPS AND HINTS FOR EXECUCIZING

This program is unusually simple to follow, but there are ways to make it even more so. By making the program even simpler, you also add to your enjoyment. Clothing is probably the first thing that comes to mind because like anything that becomes popular, exercise has developed its own fashions. You've probably heard that the only way to get anything out of a physical fitness program is to exercise while wearing tights, a "sweat suit" rubber outfit, or shorts. This is not so. Actually, sweat suits and rubber outfits should *never* be worn while execucizing because they allow the body to dehydrate. While dehydration is always dangerous, in extreme cases it can cause death. On the other hand, tights, shorts, and other styles of informal clothing are quite suitable for exercise but are not practical for office wear. And they are not all that

TIPS AND HINTS FOR EXECUCIZING

necessary for a program like execucize either. These special outfits really have only two advantages—they allow free motion, and they keep your street clothes wrinkle-free. You can have both advantages with conventional business wear. What you wear to get into shape *is not* important. For execucize, take off your jacket, loosen your tie, and roll up your sleeves whenever you can. By doing this, you give yourself the benefits of free motion. Fortunately, too, most companies allow their executives to shed jackets and ties. Only a few insist that employees be "perfectly" and correctly attired during office hours. If you work for such a company, you can still make use of execucize. After all, you can remove the jacket and loosen the tie behind your office door. It only takes a minute or two to get "neated" up when someone comes by to see you. With today's modern fabrics, you will not have to worry about wrinkling the clothes you are wearing either. If you sit down, stand up, or walk around in a business suit and do not pay attention as to whether or not it is being wrinkled, you can execucize in it.

Another thing to keep in mind, though, take your shoes off whenever you can. Being in your stocking feet makes it easier for you to do the various leg exercises because the weight of the shoes is gone. This suggestion, I must admit, usually meets with resistence. "You expect me, the vice-president of marketing, to sit at my desk in my stocking feet?" one associate of mine demanded. Another fellow looked shocked and announced, "I'm just a junior executive still trying to make a good impression. I can't be caught like that! What would I say

EXECU-CIZE

if someone saw me?" The only answer I can give to these questions is: Don't worry about having to explain to anyone why you took your shoes off. While you are sitting at your desk, no one will notice unless your business associates make a habit of crawling around under your desk while talking to you. People who stop by your office in the course of the day come to see you and not your feet. And should someone pop in while you are putting your shoes back on, there is still no problem. You can always say that you're tightening the laces, which is a common enough activity.

Now that the question of clothing is out of the way, there is the matter of air temperature to consider. The air temperature should be neither too hot nor too cold. Unusually high temperatures cause someone who is exercising to sweat too much, and the opposite, unusually cold temperatures cause people to tighten their muscles. When this happens, exercising becomes difficult; the muscles, being in a tense state, are exposed to unnecessary friction. Generally the modern office building comes equipped with central heating and air-conditioning and individuals cannot adjust the temperature to suit themselves. I have found, though, that buildings with a central thermostat are maintained at a steady and so-called comfortable temperature of about 72°. This is appropriate for exercise—it is neither too hot nor too cold. For those of you who spend your working hours in an office where the temperatures are too extreme (anything above or below 72°) try to compensate whenever possible. Opening a window slightly will

TIPS AND HINTS FOR EXECUCIZING

usually solve the problem. The outside air will either warm or cool the room. If the windows are sealed, adjust your exercise schedule. During the very cold weather, stop exercising about thirty minutes before you plan to leave the building so that your body will not be too "warm" when it is exposed to cold air. During the very hot weather, wait, again, about thirty minutes after you have come into the air-conditioned environment so that your body can adjust itself gradually to the chilly air. If you are fortunate enough to have your own thermostat, make use of it. Keep your office at 72°, the comfortable temperature for us humans. Another topic that comes up frequently during discussions about exercise is breathing.

For some reason, breathing is often a problem for people while exercising. Usually, they are inclined to hold their breath. The logic seems to be, "The human body really cannot do two things at the same time," or "Breathing interferes with exercise." Nonsense! The human body is perfectly able to do more than two things at the same time. As you read this book, you are breathing, blood is being pumped through your veins, and the last meal you ate is being processed. And these are only a few of the things that are taking place. And if your breathing does interfere with your exercising, then there is either something wrong with your respiratory system or you are not doing the exercises properly. Check your technique first. Chances are that *you* are holding your breath for no reason or that you are moving your body the wrong way and restricting your breathing. If you believe that you are performing the

EXECU-CIZE

exercises as they should be done but are still breathing with difficulty, then make an appointment with your physician to examine your respiratory system.

There are no special breathing techniques (except where otherwise noted) required for execucizing. Breathe as you would normally. By that, I mean *do not* hold your breath. Just inhale and exhale in your usual manner. Your body will adjust the respiratory system by itself should it become necessary. The harder you exercise, the more deeply, strongly, and rapidly you will breathe. Your respiratory system automatically adjusts itself to your increased oxygen needs with no conscious effort on your part. It may take you a few days to break the habit, if you are inclined to hold your breath while exercising. The best way to do this is by making a conscious effort to breathe normally while you do each execucize.

When you have completed each execucize, take a *short* rest before starting another one. For example, if you rotate your left arm counter-clockwise five times, make a pause before beginning to rotate your arm clockwise. Pause again before beginninng to rotate your right arm. Most people find thirty seconds long enough for a rest period especially for motions like those found in execucize which are not strenuous.

If, however, you feel you need a longer rest period, by all means take it. Limit your rest time to no more than a minute whenever you can. I realize that this is not always possible; the average business day does not break down so neatly. There will be occasions when you execucize in comparative peace and quiet. More than

TIPS AND HINTS FOR EXECUCIZING

likely, though, you will no sooner start an exercise sequence when you will be interrupted.

Do not let this fact worry or discourage you. There is no one perfect time for exercise. Motions that you do in the morning are just as beneficial as those you do in the afternoon. I know "regularity" is a word often heard in connection with a physical fitness program. "Put yourself on a schedule and stick to it," experts advise in their strongest voice. Excellent advice for those who are able to make their own time. Such a luxury is rarely, if ever, available to the business executive. So long as you do some execucizes each day, you are following a regular schedule. Give your muscles a work out at times that are convenient to you. As I mentioned, execucize is not a strenuous program and you can make your own schedule; I also advised you rest for thirty to sixty seconds between motions—that should be sufficient rest. Should you find that you are tired after doing an execucize, do not attempt any others until you have seen a physician. By "tired" I mean heavy breathing, sweatiness, dizziness, a need to lie down. Any such symptom is an abnormal reaction and should be discussed with a physician.

Even when you do not exhibit these symptoms, there are times when you should not exercise. Right after eating, particularly if you have had a heavy meal, is one. Give yourself at least an hour if you have eaten a light meal and an hour and a half to two hours if you have had a heavy one. If you exercise when your stomach is full, as it will be after a meal, you run the chance of developing stomach pains, cramps, or other discomforts. Over the past few years, a lot of people have been

EXECU-CIZE

ignoring this advice, and dismissing it as an "Old Wives Tale." There is a perfectly sound, scientific principle behind this caution. When your stomach is full, blood goes to your digestive organs to help them with their work. If you exert yourself physically at such a time, this blood will be drawn away from your digestive organs to your working muscles, thereby hindering or suspending digestion. None of the exercises described in this book can be classed as strenuous, but some would be difficult to perform on a full stomach. Among these are the pelvic thrusts, the abdominal exercises, and the various trunk-bending exercises. Therefore it would be wise to wait for an hour or so after eating before doing any of the motions.

Another time is when you are not feeling well. Very few executives willingly stay home when they are under the weather so if you are feeling a bit out of sorts, concentrate on getting well. Shaking off a low-grade fever, a slight head cold, or any other minor ailment should be your prime consideration.

As to actually starting, bear this essential point in mind so that your fitness program will go as smoothly as possible. Work into your program gradually. Follow the plan as it is explained because when an individual has neglected his or her body for a period of several years, a lot more damage can be done by plunging into a program of exercise without making some advance preparations. Exercise, of itself, is not dangerous, but then neither is electricity when you handle it by observing a few basic precautions. After all, you would not plug in your toaster if the cord was frayed, and you were

TIPS AND HINTS FOR EXECUCIZING

standing in a puddle of water. The same common sense holds true for exercise.

Sudden, excessive exertion after a long period of inactivity or sickness is to be avoided. If you are recovering from a major illness or operation, speak to your doctor before you start to execucize! Chances are that you will receive permission to follow a program of execucize. Even a severely damaged body can benefit from appropriate exercise. It is only when the physical activity is sudden and strenuous that harm can occur—to a healthy as well as an unhealthy individual. Anyone, though, no matter of what age or level of fitness, who suspects that there is something wrong with his heart or blood pressure should see a doctor. (For more information on this subject, see Chapter 4.) That is only common sense. And if you are over the age of *thirty*, it is particularly important that you work into the program gradually. You must prepare your body for the core of the program, and the best way to do this is to keep two things in mind: (1) your age and (2) your present level of fitness. The older you are and the lower your level of physical fitness, naturally the weaker your muscles. To skip the warm-up part of execucize is to invite pulled or torn muscles.

There will be, however, a certain amount of minor soreness which is normal after a long period of inactivity. Minor soreness and/or stiffness is caused by an accumulation of waste products within the muscles; when the waste products are cleared away, the pain ceases. Usually this process takes anywhere from one hour to twenty-four (any stiffness or soreness that takes longer

EXECU-CIZE

should be investigated). To keep muscular discomfort to a minimum, execucize calls for you to start out slowly. Gentle actions are emphasized. Forceful activity comes in time. When stiffness does occur, treat it with a *cold* compress. The same goes for a pulled or torn muscle—avoid heat—although in this case, a support bandage may be required. Your doctor is in the best position to decide.

There are a few more tips that I want to give you about execucize, but these are more of a psychological nature because your state of mind has much to do with the success of the program. Positive thinking is your greatest ally.

Before you start the program, take a good, long, *objective* look at yourself. Make note of what you see. Evaluate your condition honestly. Do you really look as well as you should or you could? Chances are that the honest answer will be NO. Then picture yourself, in your mind, as you would look if you were in top physical condition. It is not a very hard thing to do at all. When people tell me that they cannot do it, I advise them to find an old photograph of themselves. One that was made when they were young and firm. Next, I have them get a recent photo of themselves and cut off the head and place it over the head of the old photo. Presto! They know immediately how they will look when their muscles are firmed up and the flab is trimmed down. Study your mental vision of yourself—or the composite photo—until you have the image firmly set. Visualize the NEW YOU often—several times a day. For those of you who have a photo—keep it in your wallet and look at it frequently.

TIPS AND HINTS FOR EXECUCIZING

As for when to start execucize—the sooner you start, the better. You can read this book and even learn the exercises perfectly. Once you have done this, then what? You can think about starting your program of execucizes. And think. And think. Of course, the more precise term for this activity is stalling around. "I'll start next Monday when I'm fresh and relaxed from the weekend," or "I'll wait until the annual sales meeting is over," or "I'll start the program right after my vacation." All good excuses on the surface, but when you really sit down to analyze them, they come out as excuses to stall and nothing else. Certainly you can postpone the start of this program until next week, next month, or even next year, but what will that get you? Nothing. Start next week instead of this week, and that works out to seven days longer than necessary that you will walk around with flabby, unattractive muscles. When you stall around and postpone, you gain nothing. Just get yourself moving. That is essential if this program is to work for you.

And once you start the program, keep at it. This start—stop—start way some people go about a physical fitness program is next to worthless. They never get anywhere. This exercise program should be as much a part of your daily routine as brushing your teeth. Make a point of doing at least five execucizes—any five—once a day. No matter how busy your day is, you will have time for five. That is not a great number. There will be days when more time is available to you. Make use of it. Naturally, not every day can or will provide you with enough time to do more than five. Avoid trying to make excuses to yourself, though, for not doing execucizes on

EXECU-CIZE

a daily basis. I know it is very easy to find reasons not to, reasons that strike you as being noble. But remember, as I mentioned before, stalling is stalling no matter what you call it or how you dress it up.

Stay aware of the fact that this is not an instant program. You will not become a perfect physical specimen in seven days or four weeks or whatever short space of time some people claim it takes. Repairing several years of neglect is NEVER an overnight process. But then nothing that is worthwhile ever is an instant success. Accept the fact that this program will take time. Therefore, do not let yourself become discouraged. Keep reminding yourself that each day you allow yourself to execucize, you are helping your muscles, and that you are one day closer to fitness. You may not be able to see the benefits, but the benefits will be accruing. Therefore, don't rush the program. Take it one day at a time. Enjoy it. It is fun!

You will do a great favor for yourself if you forget about setting a time limit. It is a great mistake to say something like, "I'll follow this program for three weeks. If nothing happens, I'll drop it." There are two things wrong with this approach. As I said before, you cannot see what is happening to your muscles. You cannot see that they are in better shape than when you started. Because of this, you have no way of judging what progress is taking place—and progress is taking place. The other reason is that this provides a way for you to stop the program. You begin to think to yourself, "only another week, and I can drop this." And that is exactly what you will do. Setting time limits can be a valuable

TIPS AND HINTS FOR EXECUCIZING

thing in the business world, but it is useless when it comes to a physical fitness program. Do yourself a big favor. Forget about time—just follow the program.

This tip is for those of you who have tried other exercise plans in the past and have dropped them for one reason or another. I find that people who have started and then stopped other physical fitness programs tend to see themselves as "exercise failures." They are convinced that no matter what they do, they will never get back into shape. Whether consciously or unconsciously, they view themselves in terms of, "I guess I was meant to be a sagging slob. Why fight it?" Nobody is meant to be anything but what they want to be. That is my basic philosophy. If you do not like the present condition of your body, or even if you like it and want to keep it that way, you have an excellent chance of achieving your goal. There is no reason for you to dwell on your so-called past failures. Doing that is not the way to success. Telling yourself that, "I can do it," is, however, an excellent way to achieve what you want for yourself. What happened last month or last year when you started a shape-up program has absolutely no bearing on this program. Encourage yourself, praise yourself for each business day that you execucize. A personal backpat is great fodder for the ego!

And while you are indulging in self-praise, keep it personal—compare you to you. Quite often, a group of business colleagues will start an execucize program together. (For more on this subject, see Chapter 15.) I personally like this idea in principle. When I am asked about this sort of scheme, however, I do point out one

EXECU-CIZE

very important thing. No two people are ever exactly alike. On the surface, this seems like a fairly obvious, and therefore, unnecessary point to make. Actually, it is not. We tend to overlook the obvious. If you do wish to work as part of a group—fine. But if you do, do not let yourself be tempted into comparing your progress, with the progress (real or imagined) that someone else is making. This practice is almost always self-defeating. I don't know how many times I have heard something like, "Look at Charlie Jackson. He started execucizing the same time I did. His sagging stomach is all but gone. What have I got to show for my efforts?" My answer to something like that is, "Great for Charlie Jackson. But what does that have to do with you? Did you start out with a stomach that was hanging somewhere around your knees?" What someone else achieves from a physical fitness program is their business. What you achieve is yours. And by the same token, there is no need to brag to others about what you are getting out of the program. Encouraging them is one thing. Telling them you are doing better than they are is something else again. If you are really in the mood to brag, you are your own best audience. Brag to yourself. You, at least, will never lose interest in what you are doing!

If you are involved in some other fitness program or are able to participate in some sporting activity on a regular basis, don't drop it just because you have started execucize. This program is not only a solid basic program, but it can also be used as a supplement to another program. There is no such thing as too much exercise. Whatever chances come your way, take advantage of

TIPS AND HINTS FOR EXECUCIZING

them. You will be that much better off for it; you will be back in shape that much sooner.

And finally, always remember that you have a right to good health. It is not unusual for me to hear, "I put a very low priority on physical fitness. There are just too many other things I have to think about, things that are more important than whether or not my stomach hangs over my belt." Being in good shape is not something that should be treated casually. It is important; it is a gift that you can give to yourself. Teach yourself to think of a physical fitness program in those terms.

The last thing I want to tell you about so that execucize will be as successful for you as it has for so many other people, is that you ought to believe in what you are doing. Getting started is not all that hard; sticking to your resolution, that can be the hard part. For exercise to be beneficial, you need not spend an hour a day, nor do you have to suffer through countless body motions. But you do need the right ones. And you do need to do them regularly, ideally, every day. Execucize allows you to.

You also need persistence. Start. Stop. Start again. This gets you nowhere. And your poor body gets its signals crossed. Spending even a few minutes a day, but every day, regularly, is bound to show results. So believe in what you are doing. In the end, it is all a matter of believing in yourself and your abilities to get things done. That is the way to shape up to a better you.

CHAPTER 7

THE CORE EXERCISES

The Execucize Program is in three parts. There is a two-week Beginner's Program which calls for no more than three core exercises to be done no more than once a day, and the Advanced Program which calls for a *minimum* of five core exercises to be done *at least* once a day, and the Maintenance Program which is a modified version of the Beginner's Program. Sample programs and their assorted options are given in Chapter 12. Certain exercises, such as the General Body Action described below, are required during all phases of Execucize and so are not counted as being core exercises. In succeeding chapters, I will describe a number of other exercises that serve as required supplements to the core action. The core exercises are broken down into three groups: (1) Waist Exercises, (2) Waist and Leg Exercies, and (3) Leg Exercises. In each case, while performing an action, keep your stomach pulled in as far as you can. When you first

THE CORE EXERCISES

begin the program, you will, no doubt, find that you cannot pull your stomach in all that far. As you proceed, you will, however, find that your abdominal muscles are becoming stronger and firmer. This will allow you to pull these muscles in quite far and keep them there. By the way, the very act of pulling in your abdominal muscles, is, of itself, an exercise; and a fine one at that. Make it a point to tug in your stomach whenever you think of it, not just when execucizing. One other point. Many of these exercises are designed to be done while sitting in a chair. Before you start, check to see that your swivel chair is in good condition. No loose castors and what have you. If the castors are loose or the balance is poor, have repairs made.

General Body Action: This exercise is to be done before doing any other execucize described in this section. It is an all-around general muscle firmer. It serves to "warm-up" your body for your daily routine of Execucize. Stand at your desk with your back straight. Place your hands, palms down, on your desk. Do not bend your arms at the elbows. Tighten the muscles of your body and then raise yourself off the floor (no more than an inch or two) by using your arms. For the first week of the execucize program, remain in this position for a count of one only. During the second week, remain in this position for a count of two only. After the second week, you can hold this position for as long as you are able. Do not, however, exceed a count of five. Lower your body back to the floor. Release the tension on your muscles.

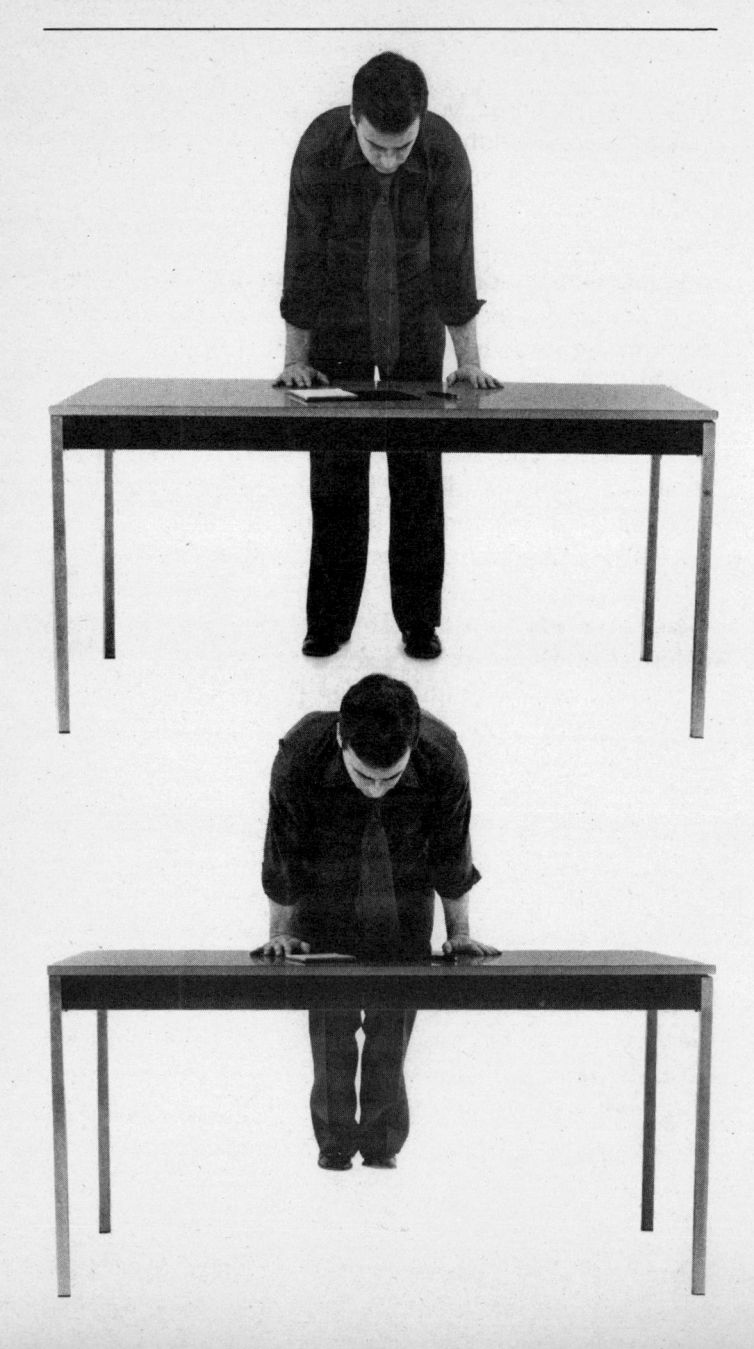

EXECU-CIZE

THE CORE EXERCISES

Execucizes For Your Waist

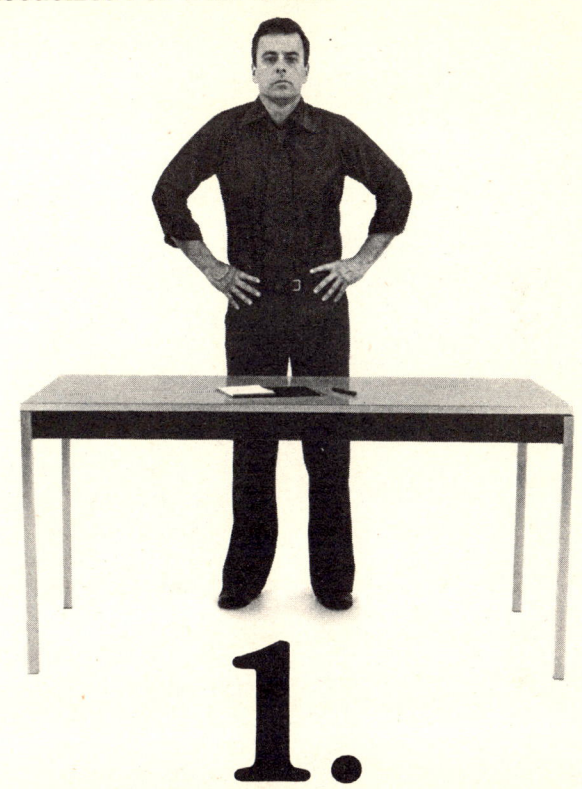

1.

Stand up straight with your legs slightly apart. Place your hands on your hips. Bend forward from your waist to a count of three. Straighten up. Bend to your right to a count of three. Straighten up. Bend to your left to a count of three. Straighten up. Bend backwards to a count of three. Straighten up. Do

59

EXECU-CIZE

this exercise only once. The action should be done with a slight jerk.

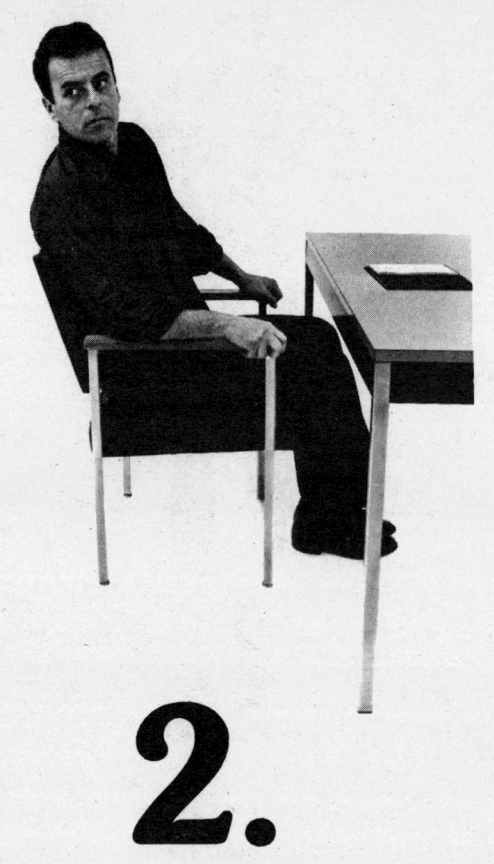

2.

Sit in your chair with your back straight. Place your feet flat on the floor and put them together. Bend your elbows and rest your arms on the arms of your chair. Grip the arms with your fingers.

THE CORE EXERCISES

Do a half-turn to your right. As you make the turn, raise your left arm slightly. This will give you leverage. And, too, turn your head in the same direction as your body. Hold this position for a count of five and return to your original position. Turn to your left in exactly the same manner and for the same count. Repeat the entire action two more times. For a variation on this motion, instead of resting your arms, extend them straight out from your sides and then execute the half-turns. The count remains the same.

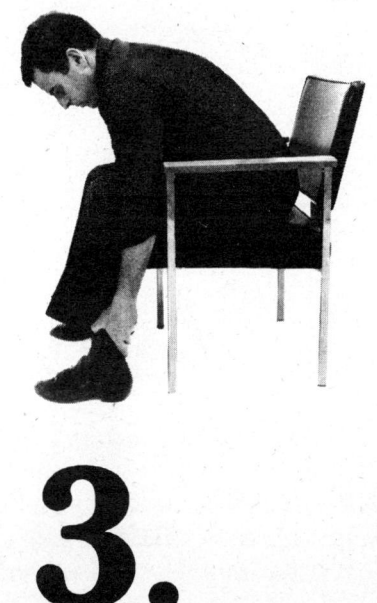

3. Sit up straight in your chair. Place your feet together and flat on the floor. Move your feet apart three paces. Drop your arms toward the floor.

EXECU-CIZE

Bend forward from your waist. Grasp your ankles from behind with your hands. Hold this position for a count of five. Return to your starting position. Repeat the entire action two more times.

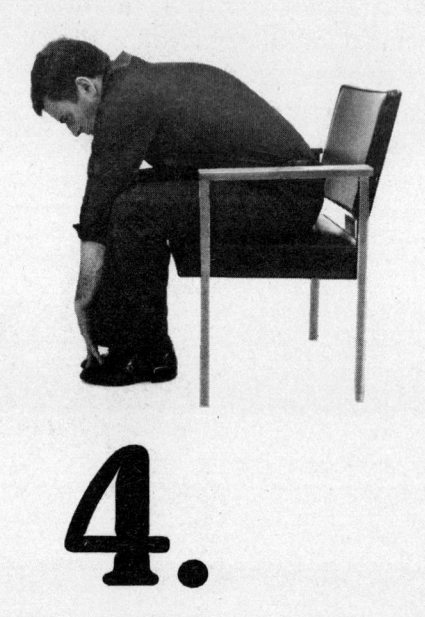

4.

Move your chair back from your desk at least three feet. Sit up straight in your chair. Place your feet flat on the floor and put them together. Bend forward from the waist and touch your toes. Hold this position for a count of five and return to your starting position. Repeat the action two more times. For a variation on this action, move your legs apart about twelve inches and then bend forward to touch your toes. The count remains the same.

THE CORE EXERCISES

5.

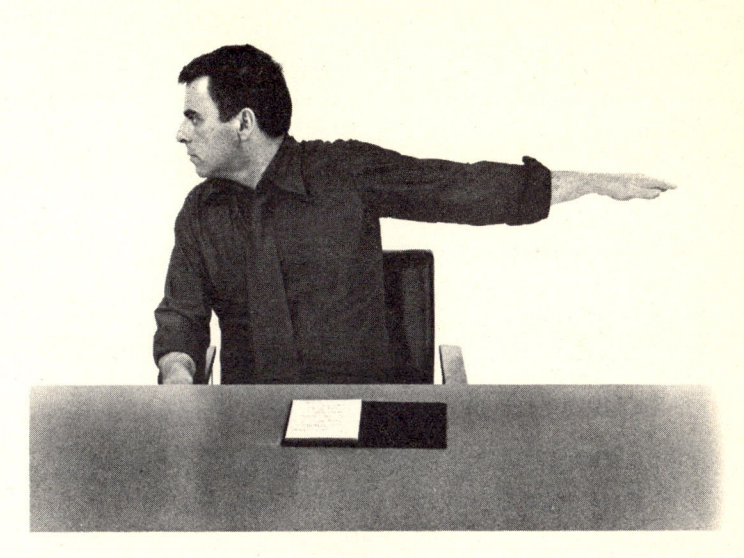

Sit up straight in your chair. Place your feet together and flat on the floor in front of you. Rest your arms lightly on the arms of your chair. Raise your left arm off the rest and extend it sideways. Do not bend your elbow. As you do this, bend toward your right side (while keeping your right arm down). Return to your original position and repeat the action, this time raising your right arm and bending toward your left. Bend in each direction five times. For a variation on this action, extend your arms straight out to your sides. Bend to your right five times and to your left five times.

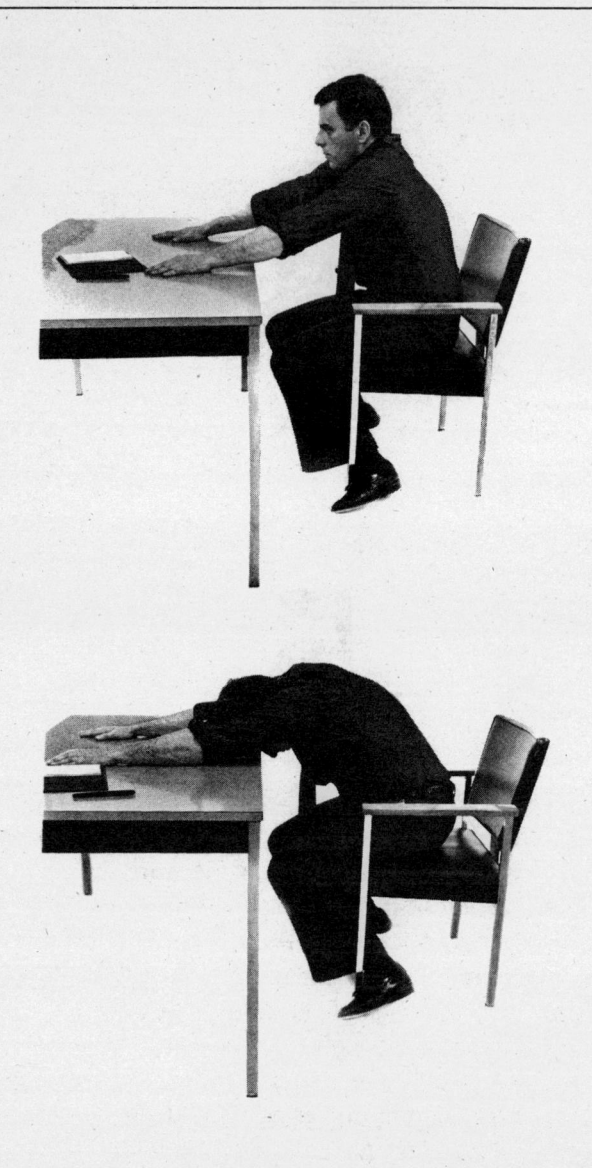

EXECU-CIZE

THE CORE EXERCISES

6.

Push your chair back about a foot from your desk. Hook your feet around the legs of your chair. Place your hands, palms down, on your desk. If your elbows are bent, then you are too close to your desk. Move back until your arms are straight. Bend forward from your waist until your forehead touches your desk. Hold this position for a count of five and return to your original position. Repeat this action four more times.

Execucizes For Your Waist And Legs: These execucizes do double-duty because two problem areas are brought into play at the same time.

EXECU-CIZE

1.

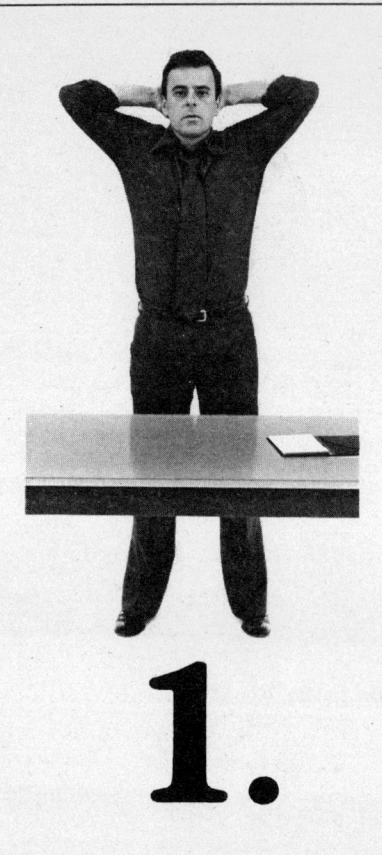

Stand straight with your legs slightly apart. Place your hands behind your neck and lace your fingers together. Tighten the muscles in your legs. Bend forward from your waist. Hold this position for a count of three. Return to your starting position. Repeat this action four more times. During the first two weeks you are execucizing, move slowly. After that, pick up speed.

THE CORE EXERCISES

2.

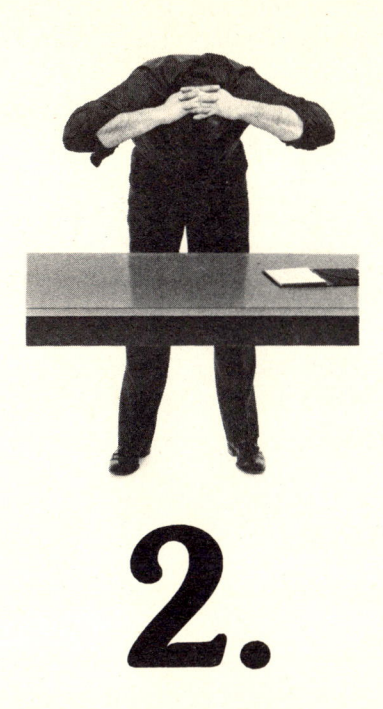

Open the bottom drawer of your desk. Move your chair so that you are able to rest your feet on the open drawer. Your legs should be straight, not bent at the knees. Position your body so that you are sitting straight in your chair. Bend forward from your waist and touch your toes while keeping your arms straight. Do not bend them at the elbows. Hold this position for a count of five and return to your starting position. Repeat the action four more times. (At the beginning of your Execucize Program, you will be able to

EXECU-CIZE

feel the muscles in your thighs pulling. Unless this is very painful and uncomfortable, do not worry about it. This "pulling" sensation merely indicates that your muscles are unaccustomed to stretching.

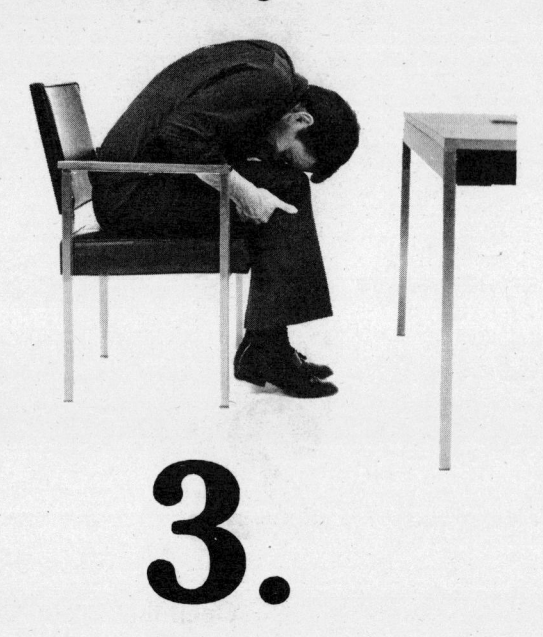

3.

While sitting straight in your chair, push it back about three feet from your desk. Place your feet flat on the floor and put them together. Place your hands behind your knees and lace your fingers together. Bend forward from your waist until your chest is resting on your knees. Hold this position for a count of five. Sit up, but keep your fingers behind your knees. Repeat the action four more times.

THE CORE EXERCISES

4.

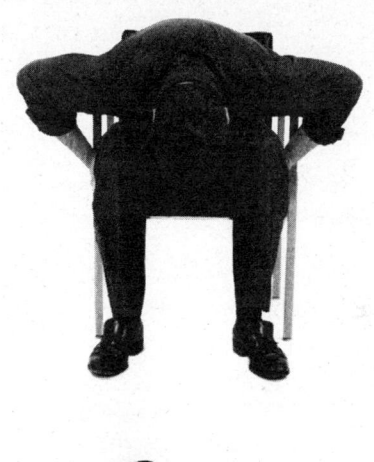

While sitting straight in your chair, push it back about three feet from your desk. Move your legs apart. Point your toes out slightly. Place your left hand behind your left knee and your right hand behind your right knee. Bend forward from your waist until your head is between your knees. Hold this position for a count of five. Sit up straight while keeping your hands behind your knees. Repeat the same action four more times.

EXECU-CIZE

5.

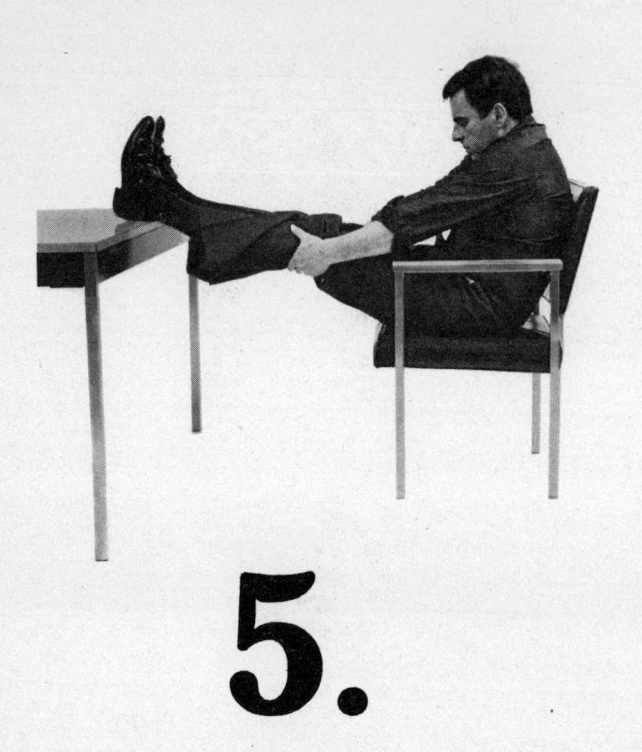

Move your chair back far enough so that you are able to rest your feet up on your desk. Your legs should be straight. Bend forward from your waist until you are able to lace your fingers behind your knees. Hold this position for a count of five. Return to your starting position. Repeat the action four more times.

THE CORE EXERCISES

6.

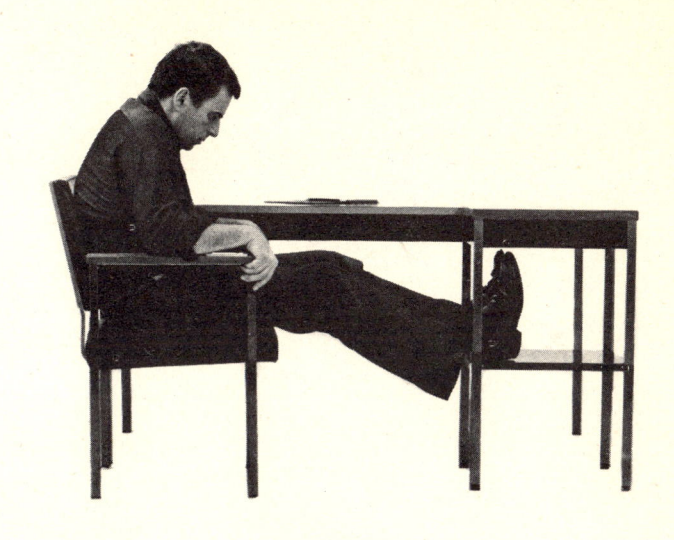

Open the bottom drawer of your desk. Move your chair so that you are able to rest your feet on the open drawer. Place your feet together and push your chair back far enough so that your knees are not bent. Rest your arms on the arms rests of your chair. Using your feet, pull yourself forward until your knees are bent; at the same time, bend slightly forward from your waist. Hold for a count of five. Push yourself back until you achieve your starting position. Repeat this action two more times.

EXECU-CIZE

7.

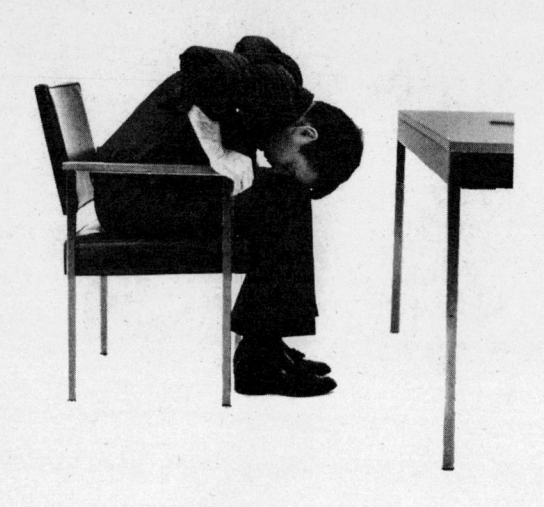

Move your chair about three feet back from your desk and sit straight. Bend forward from your waist until your head is resting on your knees. Clasp your hands behind your right knee. Sit up straight; as you are doing so, raise your leg so that it is extended out and is supported by your hands. Hold this position for a count of five. Lower your leg. Repeat the procedure with your left leg. Do this exercise only once. (When you first begin doing this exercise, you may not be able to bend all the way down to your knees or to raise your ankles up very high. Do not let this disturb you. As time

THE CORE EXERCISES

passes, and you become more supple, you will have no trouble performing this action.)

Legs

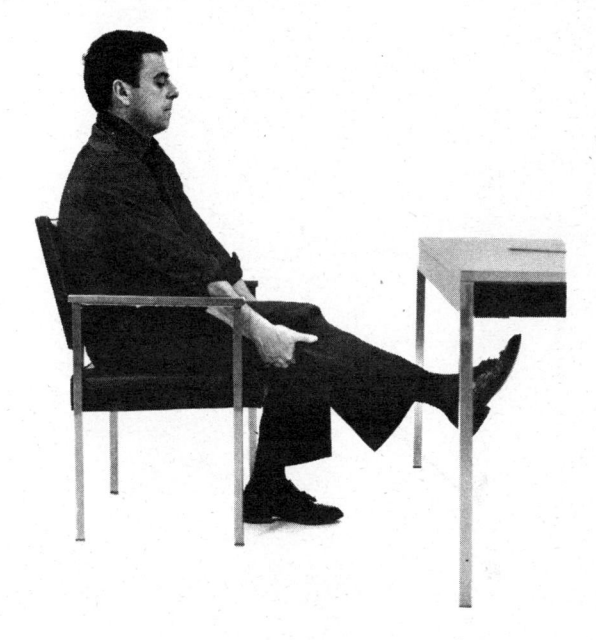

EXECU-CIZE

1.

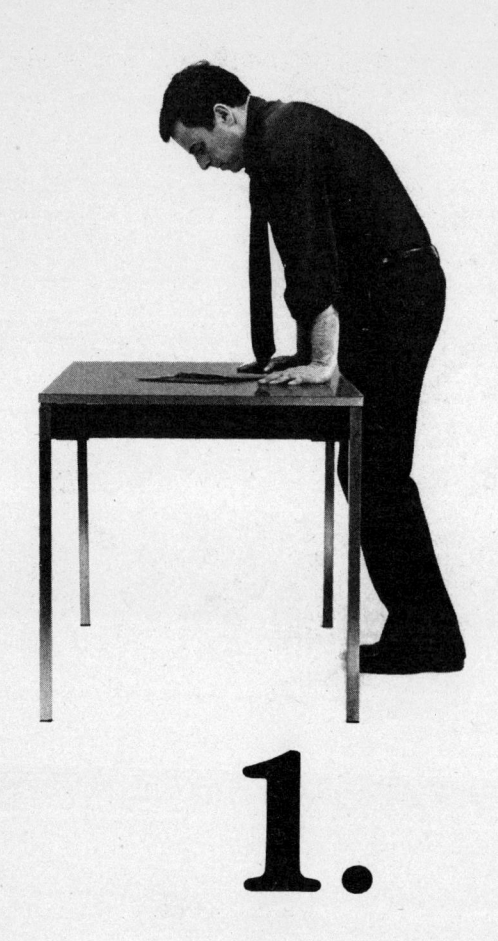

Stand facing your desk but about three inches back, with your legs together and your feet pointed slightly out. Place your hands, palms down, on your desk. Bend your knees slightly and push your pelvic section forward until it touches your desk.

THE CORE EXERCISES

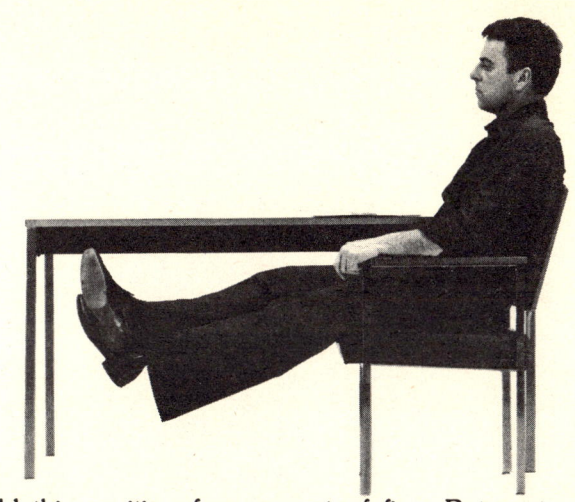

Hold this position for a count of five. Return to your starting position. Repeat the action four more times.

2.

Extend your legs straight out in front of you. Place your right ankle over your left one. Raise your legs up to a count of five. Lower them to a count of five. Repeat this action three more times. Recross your ankles so that your left ankle is over your right one. Again, raise your legs to a count of five and lower them to the same count.

EXECU-CIZE

3.

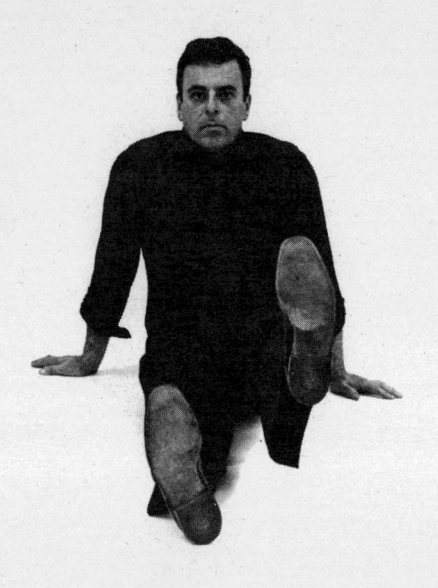

Extend one leg straight out in front of you. Rotate the leg clockwise five times and then counter-clockwise five times. Lower your leg to the floor, raise the other one, and repeat the action. Do this exercise only once. During the first two weeks of the program, rotate your leg slowly. After that, increase your speed until you are able to rotate your leg quickly. The action itself should come from the thighs.

THE CORE EXERCISES

4.

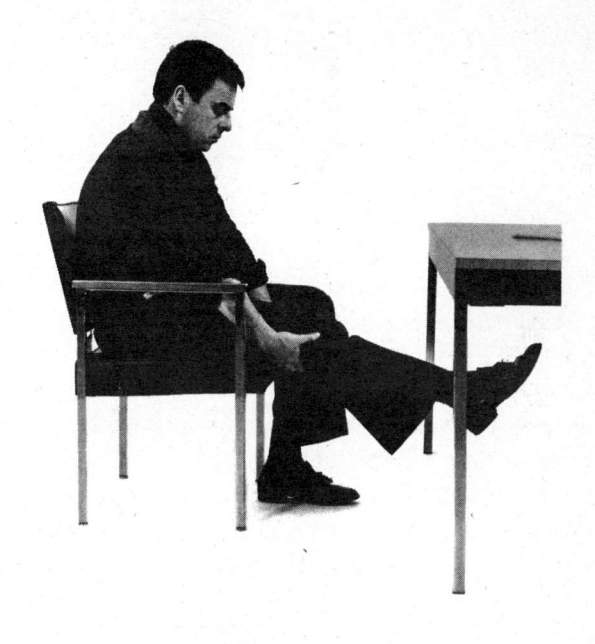

Raise your right leg off the floor and lace your fingers together behind the knee. Kick your leg out five times. Lower your right leg to the floor and raise up your left leg. Lace your fingers together behind the knee. Kick your left leg out five times. Do this exercise only once. The action should always come from your knee joint.

EXECU-CIZE

5.

Put the soles of your feet together. This will force your knees apart. Raise your feet off the floor a few inches. Swing your feet out and back. Five times out and five times back. When you first begin doing this exercise, you will feel a definite pull in the muscles of your calves and your thighs. Unless this "pulling" sensation is very painful or uncomfortable, do not let it disturb you. It is happening because these muscles are not accustomed to stretching. During the first two weeks that you are on the Execucize Program, swing slowly. After that, increase your speed so that you can do this exercise quickly.

6.

Starting out by placing your feet flat on the floor and slightly apart. Lift your feet off the floor about four inches and then move them up and down as though you were pedaling a bicycle. Keep this action up for a count of ten. During the first two weeks that you are following the Execucize Program, pedal

THE CORE EXERCISES

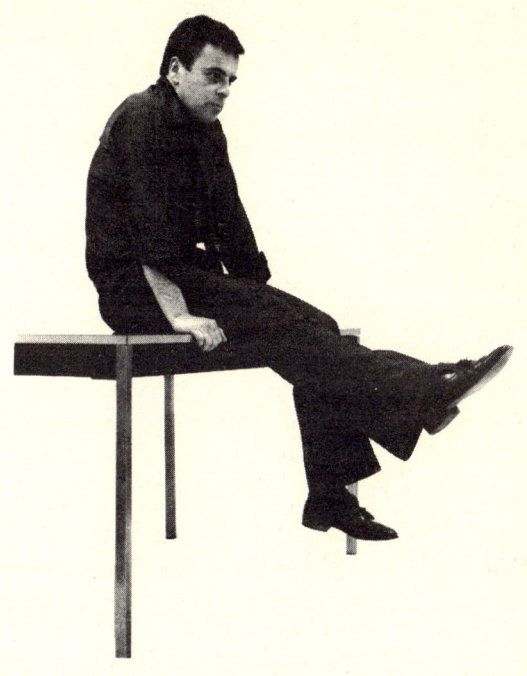

slowly. After that, gradually increase your speed until you are able to move your feet at fairly good clip.

7.

This action is ideal for those times when you are using a dictating machine. Sit on your desk so that your legs dangle in front of the chair

EXECU-CIZE

opening. Put your feet together and kick them out for a count of ten. Bring your legs to a stop. Kick your right leg out five times and then your left leg. During the first two weeks of your Execucize Program, kick slowly. After that, increase your speed so that you are able kick your leg very fast.

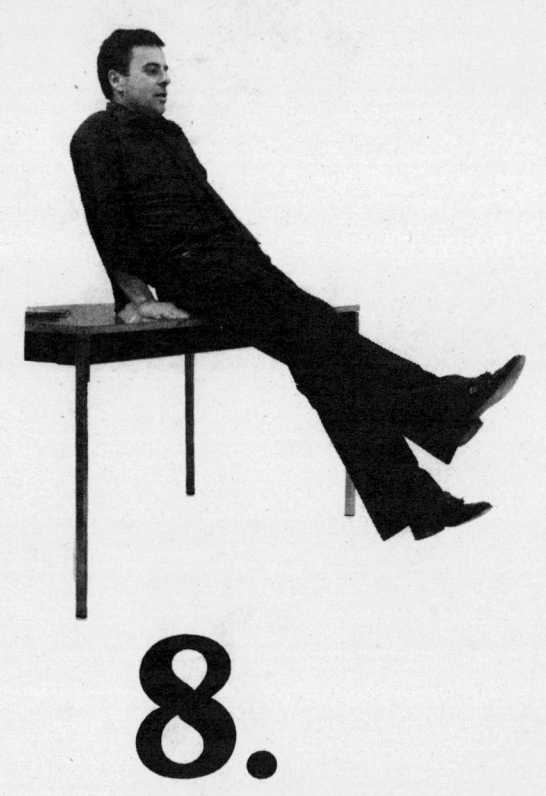

8.

Again, sit on your desk. Bring your buttocks as close to the edge as possible.

THE CORE EXERCISES

Lean back slightly and support your weight by placing your hands, palms down, on your desk. Extend your legs straight out in front of you. Kick them up and down as though you were swimming. Continue this action for a count of ten. Do this exercise only once. During the first two weeks of the program, kick slowly. After that, increase your speed so that you are able to kick faster and faster.

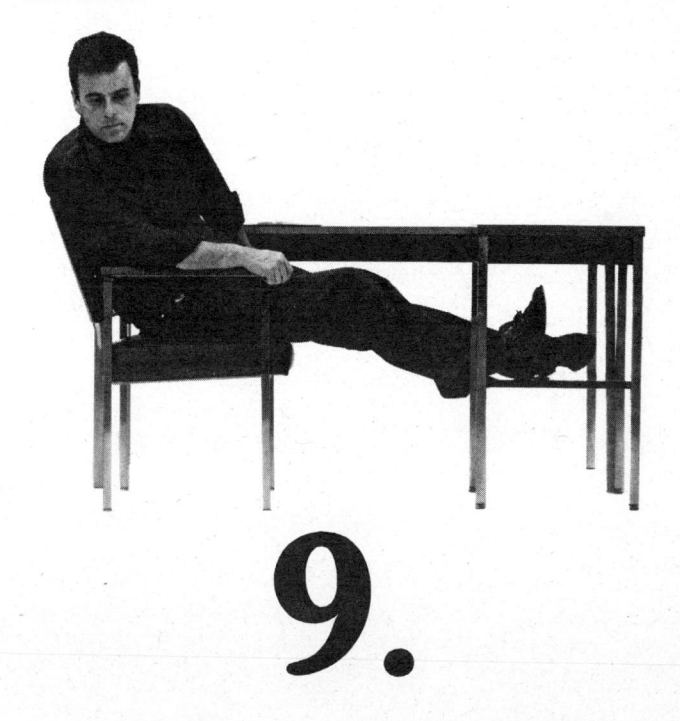

9.

Open the bottom drawer of your desk. Move your chair so that you are able to rest your feet on the drawer. With your hands lightly grasping

EXECU-CIZE

the arm rests of your chair, roll on your right hip toward your right. Roll on your left hip toward your left. Return to your starting position. Repeat the entire sequence four more times. Your legs should be extended straight—your knees should not be bent.

10.

Grasp the arms of your chair firmly with your hands. Extend your legs straight out in front of you. Open and close them as though they were a pair of scissors. Continue this action for a count of ten. A variation on this action is to cross and recross your legs at the ankles. This action is also maintained for a count of ten. During the first two weeks of the Execucize Program, do both of these actions slowly. After that, increase your speed until you can do them rapidly.

THE CORE EXERCISES

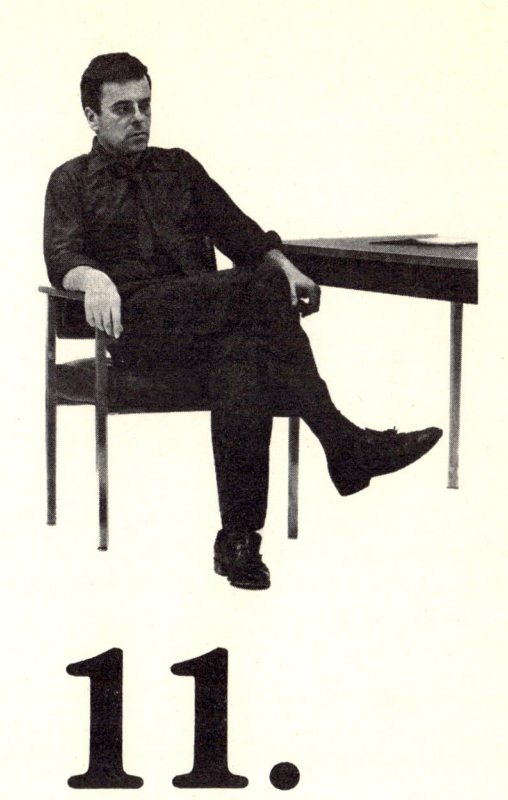

11.

Place your feet flat on the floor. Cross and recross your legs over your thighs. Your right leg goes over your left leg five times and your left over your right five times. Do this exercise only once. A variation is to cross and recross your ankles. For the ankle-cross, the count is also ten. The starting position, as well, is the same. During the first two weeks of the Execucize Program, the crossing action, whether of your

EXECU-CIZE

legs or your ankles, should be done slowly. After that, increase your speed so that you are doing this action as rapidly as possible.

Now that we have covered the "core" exercises, it is time to move on to the ones that serve as supplements.

CHAPTER 8

GOOD MORNING, GOOD EVENING

When you arrive at the office each morning, what do you do? "Get right to work," you are probably thinking as you read this. And I don't doubt that you do, not for one second. But how do you get down to work? If you are anything like I was, you probably behave something like the fellow in this little scenario. Mr. Modern Executive arrives at the office. If his secretary is at her desk, he pauses to have a quick conference with her. Then he checks over his incoming calls and mail and disappears into his office. There he hangs up his hat and coat and settles down at his desk where he opens his briefcase and pulls out the papers he needs. Without further ado, he settles down in his chair

85

EXECU-CIZE

and begins to work. While this is common behavior, you will notice that Mr. Modern Executive has done no exercise. He has moved his body around a bit, but that is all. What is more, he has passed up several opportunities for exercise. Let's go back over this scene and demonstrate how this daily entry can be turned into a valuable exercise session—one that you can use.

Mr. Modern Executive arrives at the office ready for a hard day's work and a fair amount of exercise. Let's assume that he stops at his secretary's desk for a brief conference. Let's also assume that she has papers for him. She gathers them together and hands them to him. If Mr. Modern Executive just wanted to move his body, he would position himself so that he has merely to extend his arm. There is nothing wrong with doing so, but, of course, such an action also does nothing to encourage physical fitness. The fellow who wanted to exercise would stand far enough back from his secretary's desk so that he is forced to reach forward for the papers. By doing this, our Modern Executive stretches his abdominal as well as his arm muscles. And as a further benefit, this action takes NO extra time.

Once inside his office, Mr. Modern Executive is presented with another opportunity for exercise. His briefcase is placed on the floor while he takes off his hat and coat and hangs them up. But instead of just hanging them up, Mr. Modern Executive will execucize them up like this and so can you. As you remove your hat, stand up on tiptoe (this can be done even while wearing shoes). Place your hat on the rack or shelf. Lower yourself. Remove your coat. Stand up as high as you can

GOOD MORNING, GOOD EVENING

on tip-toe and put your coat on the hanger. Lower yourself. If you take off your jacket at the same time, repeat the process. Now you are ready to retrieve your briefcase from the floor. As you reach for it, bend your knees slightly and pick it up, but not by the handle. Rather, pick it up as though it were a box of some sort. Extend your arms straight out in front of you and walk toward your desk. Put it down and open it. Another execucize to come, but how you execucize while removing the papers you need for the day, depends on what type of case you carry. If you have the attache type, move back from the desk so that you will have to stretch to reach inside. If you carry the standard briefcase type, stretch by standing up on your toes once again. Bend forward as much as you need to get at the papers.

This sequence of execucizes can be repeated when you leave the office in the evening (or anytime you leave your desk). Stretch and reach for those papers you plan to take home with you. Stretch and reach for your hat and coat. Naturally, the more you do these stretching exercises, the greater the benefits you will derive from them. There is no such thing as "too much" when it comes to stretching.

Stretching your body is a good general exercise because such an action requires you to use nearly every muscle you have in your body. It is also a good way to get a figurative "shot in the arm." You feel better, more alert and awake, afterward. And as an executive, you know how important it is to feel alert.

CHAPTER 9

GRACE UNDER PRESSURE

We are all, no matter what work we do, subject to what is known as pressure, stress, or tension. The precise word is not particularly important; the condition, however, is. Those who have white collar jobs absorb more than their share of pressure. It really cannot be helped because stress comes with the position as does the desk, the intercom, and the secretary. What can be helped is your reaction. You can learn to lessen the severity of your reaction through execucize. But before you do so, you should know what stress really is. The term is bandied about but is rarely, if ever, defined and explained. And it should be because there is stress and there is stress.

Stress is nothing more than nervous tension, and it comes in several forms. There is conscious stress. That is when you know quite well that you are under tension.

GRACE UNDER PRESSURE

There is also unconscious stress, and as the term implies, it is that which you are unaware of. There is also "environmental" and "psychological" tension. That is you may be reacting to a physical or an emotional situation. And tension may be "acute" or "chronic" whereby the source is a one time event or a continuing situation. (These are just some of the more common variables.) Stress, tension, or whatever results when you react to particular situations which, to your way of thinking, threaten or exert pressure on you. So whatever the source or the form, tension, in the end, depends on your *reaction* and not on the particular event or situation.

It is important, though, to distinguish between the types of stress. Today, it is fashionable to talk about the dangers of stress on the body. This talk, however, tends to be in vague terms that ignore the distinctions found in the area of stress. Indeed, such talk often confuses these different types even though their relationship with the body can differ greatly. It is especially important that a distinction be made between environmental and psychological stress and acute and chronic. Acute environmental stress is a passing condition. It is any incident which is unexpected and requires you to react immediately. An example might be having a tire blow out while you are driving along a highway. However unpleasant this form of tension may be, it does have one advantage—it is temporary. It goes as quickly as it comes.

Chronic environmental stress is a reaction often brought about by long-term exposure to overcrowded, noisy working and/or living conditions. This form of

EXECU-CIZE

pressure can also result from living and working in unusually isolated areas, too. Isolation as a source of stress is not as common as overcrowding. Psychological stress, though, is the more common form and the type that you are most likely to feel. While waiting to hear whether or not you will be promoted, you may undergo acute psychological tension. Once you know the decision, you at least know where you stand. The "not knowing" is the cause of your reaction. Chronic psychological stress, however, is the result of long-term dissatisfaction with something. The classic example is being stuck in a job that you cannot stand.

Along with any discussion of tension, mention is often made of The Fight or Flight Response. You may be hearing this term a lot, but I doubt very much that it has ever been explained. It is this response to stress that causes all the problems. Fight or Flight can be explained with an illustration.

Assume, for a moment, that you are driving along a quiet street. Your mind, occupied with other things, is not really on driving. Suddenly, a child darts from between two parked cars. At the very last moment, you realize what is happening and slam on the breaks. The child, quite safe, scampers off. You, however, begin to shake and breath heavily. A threat from the environment (in this case, the possibility of injuring a child) has caused a Fight or Flight reaction. Your body adjusted itself, hence the shakiness, heavy breathing, cold sweat. The reaction comes about this way.

Your brain sends out signals to stimulate the autonomic nervous system (we have no conscious control over

GRACE UNDER PRESSURE

this either). This stimulation causes the release of powerful hormones (including epinephrine) which prepare the body for action. Your body moves into high gear so that there is an increase in the rate and strength of your heartbeat, a constriction of blood vessels and a rise in your blood pressure, an increase in your blood sugar and fatty acids, a dilation of your nostrils and bronchi, an increased level of tension in your muscles, retraction of your eyeballs and the dilation of your pupils. Furthermore, the time necessary for your blood to coagulate is reduced. All these changes are necessary to speed your reactions and make you more capable of any extrordinary physical effort that the danger may require whether it is fighting or running away.

This Fight or Flight response is basic to human nature and was essential to our primitive ancestors who had to chose whether they would stay and fight the environmental threat or turn tail and run from it. Yet this reaction, however basic, is rarely appropriate to modern life. Very few environmental threats can be handled by either fighting or running. In the example I used, the child darting in front of your car, there was only one practical solution—hit the breaks and hard! What can you fight in such a situation? What can you run from? Nothing. Yet because of the automatic reaction to environmental stress, your body is left prepared for a struggle or a flight that never occurs. And because of this, certain physical alterations take place that can prove unhealthy in the long run. The release of epinephrine has caused fatty acids—needed to fuel the muscles and make the blood clot more quickly if a wound occurs—to enter your blood stream. When a struggle does not take place, these fatty acids are left circulating through the blood vessels and may then convert into cholesterol deposits. Furthermore, repeated subjection to the fight or flight response can result in permanent high blood pressure. In fact, research suggests that repeated environmental stress situations can be a major cause of atherosclerosis and other heart diseases when no extraordinary physical movement is possible to "burn" up your body's unnecessary overproduction of fatty acid. That is what acute environmental stress can do.

Chronic environmental stress, as I mentioned earlier, is living and/or working within extraordinary conditions over a long period of time. Miners, for example, frequently exhibit chronic environmental stress. Their working conditions are cramped and noisy. Every day a miner may face acute environmental stress—an accident may threaten. Even when an accident does not take place, the miner must be on the alert. The human body can adjust to chronic environmental stress. It is called the General Adaption Syndrome. This is not always a permanent solution, though. People subjected to chronic environmental stress can, and often do, develop high blood pressure and high levels of blood cholesterol. Complete physical and mental breakdowns can occur.

Psychological stress refers to the emotional effect of particular incidents. Like environmental stress, psychological tension can last for varying periods of time from a few minutes to several years.

Acute psychological stress caused by conflict can have its source in interpersonal relationships (losing an argument). The source can also be an abstract such as time (a lengthy estimate must be prepared within an hour). Whatever the source, acute psychological stress produces a reaction very similar to acute environmental stress.

There are two main sources of this type of stress—conflict and change. Both sources generally bring on the physical changes associated with the Fight or Flight reaction. The reaction itself is an automatic one, over which we can have little, if any, conscious control. But, again, the reaction tends to be physically unnecessary and so the same physically damaging effects can occur. Acute psychological stress due to change, however, involves no Fight or Flight reaction. Change, though, is psychologically stressful to many people. And the type of change does not really matter. It can be a promotion, a move to a new city, a marriage, a death. You name it. The more changes an individual must face and adapt to at once, the more likely it is that tension will appear. The usual human reaction to change is, oddly enough, illness. Just why this is so is not fully understood even by the experts. People who experience a high level of stressful change in their lives over a limited period of time (whether it be one major stressful happening or a number of small ones) usually develop some form of physical illness within a few months. One researcher questioned and tested people on their recent experiences of typical stressful events (ranging, for example, from changing one's eating habits to suffering the death of a spouse.) The top ten percent of those studied suffered twice as much physical illness in the next four months as those in the bottom ten percent.

Chronic psychological stress depends much more

EXECU-CIZE

on the individual than on what actually happens to him. It is chronic psychological tension that affects members of the business community more than any other form. For example, someone who has been promoted above his abilities will probably be under such constant stress. Of course, some individuals may not be aware of the pressure, or of not being up to the job. On the other hand, someone in a position well within his capabilities may also be under constant tension. Perhaps it is because he cannot admit to himself that he can do it easily; or because he wants to win a promotion; or simply because that is his way of doing things. This last point is particularly important.

Some heart researchers, in fact, believe that there are two distinct personality types, and they have profiled them. Type A has intense ambition, competitive drive, and a sense of urgency about everything. Type B, in constrast, has a quiet, calm personality. It takes a great deal to get a Type B personality upset. These researchers have also suggested that type A personalites are far more likely to get heart disease. As yet, though, no one has presented conclusive proof of this so the suggestion remains only a suggestion. The high correlation between the so-called "Type A" people and heart disease can be explained equally as well by higher cholesterol and blood pressure levels occurring because of other forms of stress. Nevertheless, those under chronic psychological stress do often develop some form of illness. The symptoms of stress-induced ailments can be physical, mental, or psychosomatic. By the way, psychosomatic does not necessarily mean that you are imagining your symptoms. It means rather, that you are under such

GRACE UNDER PRESSURE

chronic psychological stress that you have worked yourself into an ailment of some sort. In extreme cases, chronic psychological pressure can produce a nervous breakdown. Generally, though, the illnesses associated with chronic psycological stress are of a more common nature—asthma, indigestion, migraine, ulcers, heart palpitations. The very diseases the business man is most likely to complain of. But perhaps the most obvious symptom of psychological stress, whether acute or chronic, that the average businessman displays is temper. Probably because losing your temper is the easiest way to release the tension that has built up. Yet fussing, fuming, shouting, snapping is not the answer because your body reacts in a negative fashion. "Blowing your top" produces the same physical conditions that occur during the Fight or Flight response.

None of this presents a very pretty picture. Stress causes more problems than it ever solved. I believe very few would argue that point with me. Yet it exists and the business world has more than its share of tension. I do not have to tell you where it's at when it comes to pressure. There are always the reports that should have been ready yesterday. There is always the possibility that your best customer might be wooed away by your competitor. There are the rumors of mergers that might cost you your job. And a good many business executives even chew their nails about things over which they have no direct control; things that not even the most demanding superior can hold them responsible for. Why, in my own organization, we've been sweating the sinking dollar. As a result, tempers are rather short.

Because of all the stress, whether it comes from the

EXECU-CIZE

responsibilities of the job or from just plain, living, people react. And I find that executives generally show the signs of tension more than other people. This is not, of course, to say that no other career is subject to stress. Rather, I am saying that executives get more than their share of pressure, and they show it, too. How many of your associates have high blood pressure, heart trouble, ulcers? Maybe you yourself do. Well, my feeling is that as long as we are talking about getting you back into good physical shape, we might just as well talk about getting you back into good emotional shape. The most perfect assortment of muscles in the world will not do you much good if you let yourself be caught up in the stresses and strains that come your direction every day. Relaxing is part of being in good physical condition, too. And while you are loosening up your muscles so that you can relax, you can also tighten them up so you look better. Being able to loosen up and relax is not very difficult either. The execucizes described below are designed so that you can loosen up while firming up in the easiest possible way.

This first execucize is an all-purpose action that is great to know about and use when you are faced with an office crisis. The precise problem is not really important. But for the sake of illustration, we can say that you have been told that you must get a bid ready for your company's biggest customer by five o'clock in the afternoon. It is now eleven o'clock in the morning. You have to assemble all the information, work up the figures, check them over, and then dictate the whole thing to your secretary. You feel as though you have just

GRACE UNDER PRESSURE

been hit by a bombshell. Your first instinct is to say, "Why, that's impossible. It can't be done." But you know better. Such an excuse would be unacceptable. Impossible or not, the bid must be ready. All you can think of is the fact that there is so little time. You break out in a cold sweat. You find it difficult to think, to concentrate. There is a knot in your stomach. This is a classic example of what being under pressure can do. If you stay in this condition, you will not be able to work at your most efficient level. You are going to have to relax. Get yourself together so that you can move forward.

The first thing to do if you are to relax is to sit down at your desk. Settle into your chair with your spine straight and your shoulders squared off. Place your hands, palms down, firmly on the top of your desk. Drop your eyelids. There is no need to squeeze them shut. Just drop them as though you were preparing for sleep. Clear your mind of the problem facing you at the moment. Don't pay any attention to it for a few minutes. The problem will wait for you. If you have trouble making your mind blank, create a mental picture of something that pleases you. Something you would like to be doing at that particular moment. My favorite vision is that I am walking along an ocean beach. The day is clear, sunny and quite warm. The sound of the waves lapping against the sand is soothing; I haven't a care in the world, and all my bills are paid. Once you have your particular vision in your mind, take a deep, deep breath and hold it for a count of five. Slowly exhale. Slowly, but fully. Take another deep breath and hold it for a count of five. Exhale. Repeat this process until you feel yourself

EXECU-CIZE

relax. I find that sixty to ninety seconds of deep breathing is all that I need. As you inhale, pull your stomach muscles in as far as you can and press against your desk with your hands so that the muscles of your arms feel tight. As you exhale, release the tension on your arm muscles and let your stomach out a bit.

This deep breathing serves to increase the level of oxygen in your blood. As a result, the effects of the Fight or Flight response are neutralized; the response is stopped before it really gets going. You feel more alert, better able to concentrate. In short, you are in control of yourself, and the problem does not seem so overwhelming. You have more energy to devote toward solving the problem.

This breathing exercise is also very good for those times when the pressure builds up while you are working. Those times when fourteen people are chasing after you demanding that you accomplish eighteen assignments in twenty minutes. Those times when a small thing, like a misplaced pen, is liable to set you off. Losing your temper under such circumstances accomplishes nothing except to make you feel worse than you already do. When you feel your temper beginning to flare up, sit yourself down and take a breathing break. You will be surprised at how quickly the urge to set the sparks flying will pass. It will also serve to make you a more popular, likable individual. And you will go a long way toward earning a reputation as someone who can keep his cool under the most trying circumstances. Those who hang on tend to hang in until they reach the top!

GRACE UNDER PRESSURE

Another time when this breathing exercising is an excellent technique to use is when the pressure comes off. When the rush assignment is completed. When you are finally finished for the day and are ready to head for home. That is when I am most likely to take a breathing break. Just before I leave the office. The challenges of the business day are over, but the challenges of driving home in rush-hour traffic are about to begin. I sit down and breathe for a minute or so. It is more relaxing, I feel, than a warm shower. You can actually feel the tensions of the day slipping from your body. And at the same time, you are firming up the muslces of your stomach and your arms.

Unfortunately, there is more to being under tension than a cold sweat and a knot-like feeling in the pit of your stomach. There is also a fierce headache. The throbbing kind. The sort of headache that makes it difficult to see straight because you feel as though there is a little monster behind your eyeballs pinching them. The sort of headache that makes it difficult to think. Using your mind actually hurts. Rather than suffer with it or swallow a couple of aspirin, why not execucize the headache away along with the stress that is causing it? And while you are doing that, you will also be giving some attention to your facial muscles. This is one part of the body too often ignored during a shape-up program, yet your facial muscles need exercise as much as your stomach muscles.

These next few execucizes are for those headaches that are centered in the area of your eyes. You can use any one to soothe away your headache. First, though,

EXECU-CIZE

clear your mind of office problems; turn your thoughts to something else, anything else, that pleases you. If you wear eyeglasses, remove them.

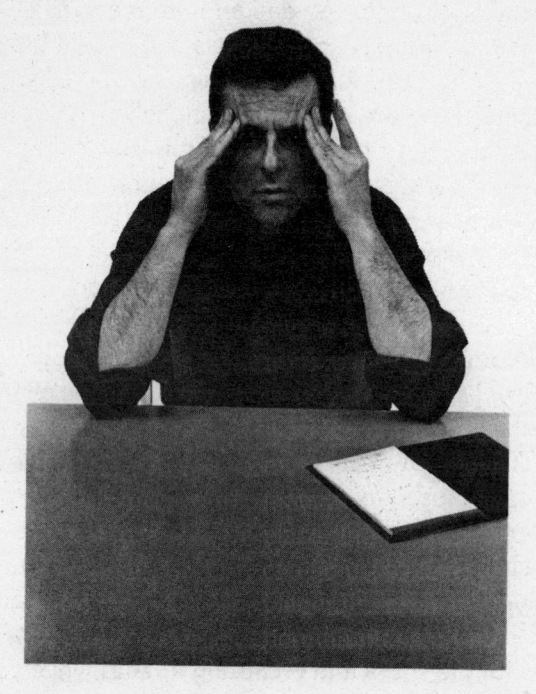

1.

Place your elbows on your desk. Drop your head forward so that your fingertips are

GRACE UNDER PRESSURE

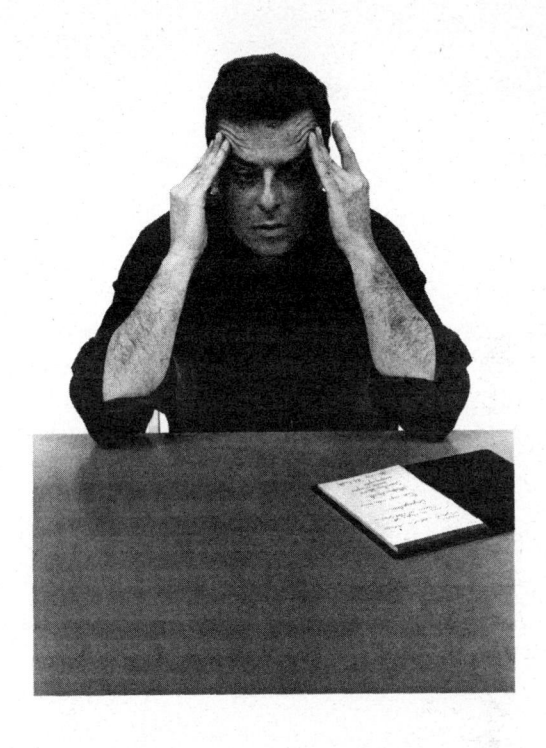

just above your eyebrows. Slowly run your fingertips along the skin until you come to the end of your brow line. Now lift the skin up gently toward your hair line. Hold this position for a count of ten and return your fingertips to your starting point. Keep this gentle and slow action up for about three minutes.

EXECU-CIZE

2.

For this execucize, place your fingertips on your temples. Again, using a gentle and slow motion, rotate the skin upward in the direction of your hair line. This is a very soothing action and takes between two and three minutes to work.

GRACE UNDER PRESSURE

3.

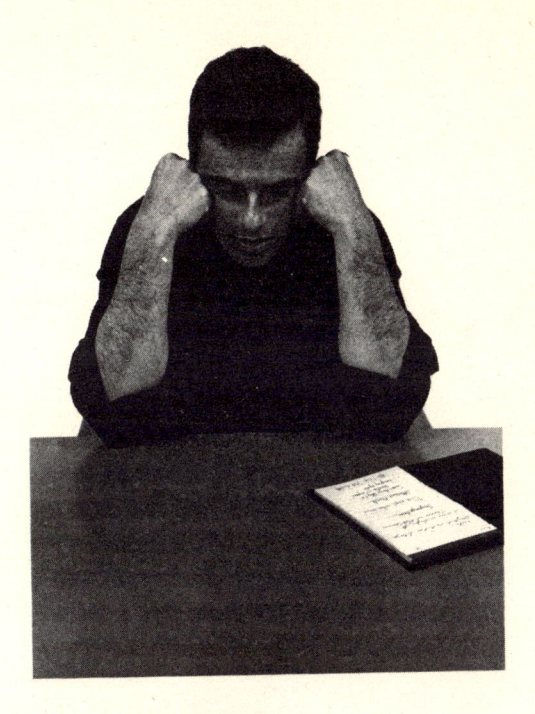

        This is a variation on the above execucize. Curve your fingers down in a claw-like manner. Rest them on your jaw line. Move your fingertips along the line of your jaw. As you do so, gently pull your skin up until you reach your temples. Once you

EXECU-CIZE

reach your temples, rotate your fingertips. Place your fingers back on your jaw line and repeat the process four more times.

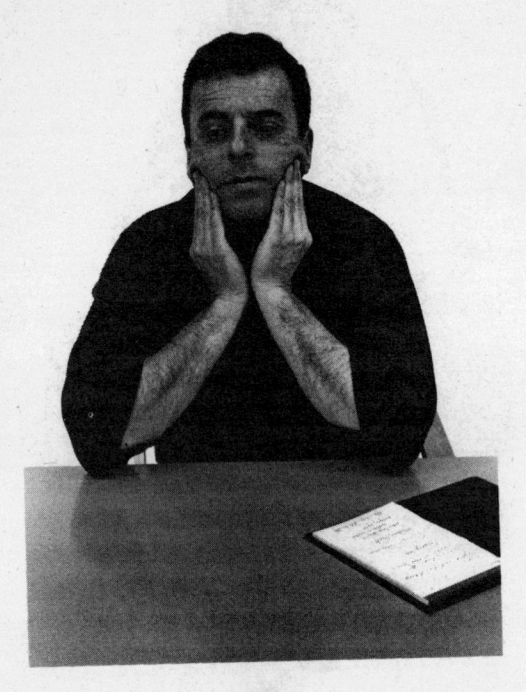

4.

Place your fingers together. Rest the tips on your jaw, on either side of your chin. Move your hands upward along your cheeks, around

GRACE UNDER PRESSURE

your eyes until you reach your hairline. As you do this, gently pull your facial skin upwards. Repeat this action five times.

This next group of execucizes, described below, works especially well on the headache centered at the back of your neck. They are designed to loosen those muscles while firming them up.

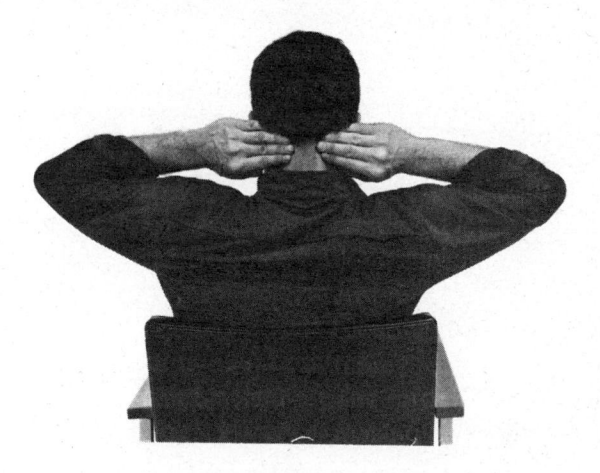

1.

Put your fingers at the nape of your neck and slowly rotate them in a clockwise direction for a count of fifteen and then reverse the

EXECU-CIZE

action so that you go in a counter clockwise direction—again, for a count of fifteen. Use a gentle pressure.

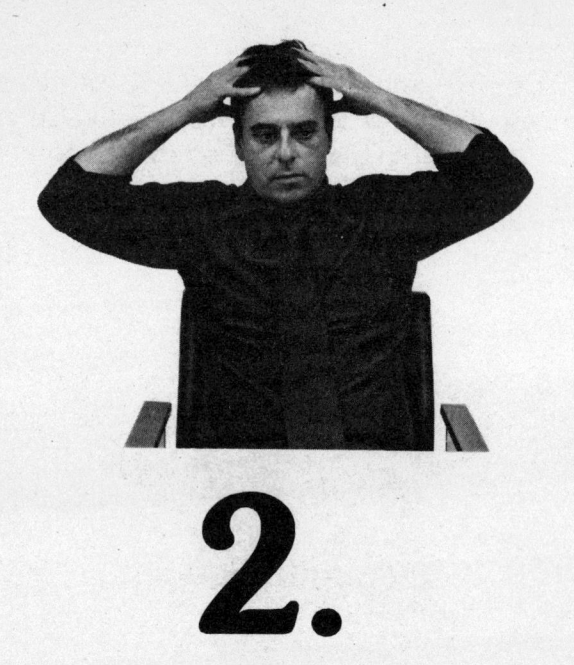

2.

Place your fingertips on your scalp, making sure that they are resting on skin and not on your hair. Using a circular motion, work your fingertips up along your scalp until you reach the top of your head. Return your fingers to your hairline and repeat the procedure two more times. (Quite often, I am asked if this action will prevent baldness or stimulate hair growth. I am sorry to say that it will not. All it will do is soothe you and firm up the muscles of your scalp.)

GRACE UNDER PRESSURE

3.

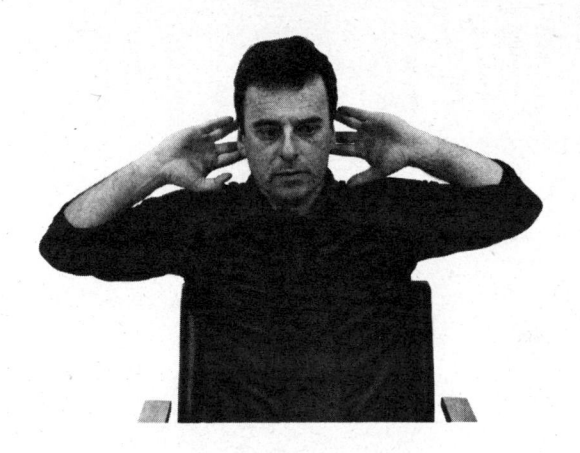

Rest your fingers behind your ear lobes. In a circular motion, work the tips up and around your ears until you reach your temples. Continue the circular motion for a count of five. Repeat this action four more times.

When you find yourself with a headache that is around *eyes and* the back of your neck, do an exercise for each area. All of these execucizes can be used as often as you like in the course of a day.

As you can see, tightening the skin around your neck and face is a great way to relax.

CHAPTER 10

WHEN THE TELEPHONE RINGS

The most annoying aspect of working in an office, I find, is the telephone. Unfortunately, this aid to modern communication has no respect whatever for the concentration so necessary to the modern executive. No sooner do you settle down with a report that absolutely has to be read and commented upon when the telephone rings. To make matters worse, it is not always possible to have your calls held. There are always people to whom you have to speak. The fact that you are busy does not enter into the situation at all. The calls that can be taken care of with a few words or even a sentence or two are bad enough, but what about those calls that drag on? The ones that last for at least five minutes, and in some cases, even longer. What can be done about them? They cannot be

WHEN THE TELEPHONE RINGS

stopped, and this fact leaves you with a choice. You can sit at your desk and listen, making an occasional comment or giving an occasional grunt to indicate that you are still listening, or more accurately, that you are still at the other end of the wire. You can also accept the fact that you are stuck on the telephone and do something for yourself until you can free yourself and get back to what you were doing. Personally, I find the telephone a nuisance, except, of course, when the shoe is on the other foot, and I have to get in touch with someone. This set of exercises came about as a result of my boredom. I was stuck on the phone one afternoon with a gabby soul who also happened to be an excellent customer. When the phone rang, I was in the middle of dictating a letter to my secretary—a letter that I wanted to go out that afternoon. My caller, after checking on some prices, launched into a discussion of how well his daughter was doing at dancing school. This five year old was showing all the signs of being the next Maria Tallchief. And you can't say to one of your best customers, "I don't give a d—m," and hang up. He had me, and to kill time, I started doing some exercises. None of these exercises are mental distractions, they can be done even while you are discussing business. The only thing is that you cannot do them if you have to write. Once you finish your notetaking, though, you can go right back to exercising, and your caller will never be the wiser. You will, however, be the better for it as you work yourself back into shape.

EXECU-CIZE

1.

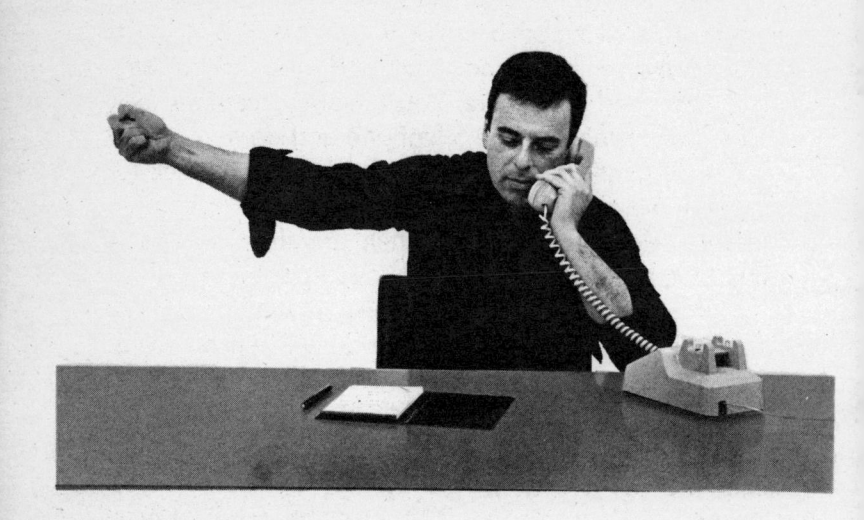

With your free hand, make a fist, a fairly tight one. For women who have long fingernails, be careful not to dig them into your hands. Extend your arm straight out and tighten the muscles. Hold this position for a count of five. Gradually release the tension. Repeat this action once more.

WHEN THE TELEPHONE RINGS

2.

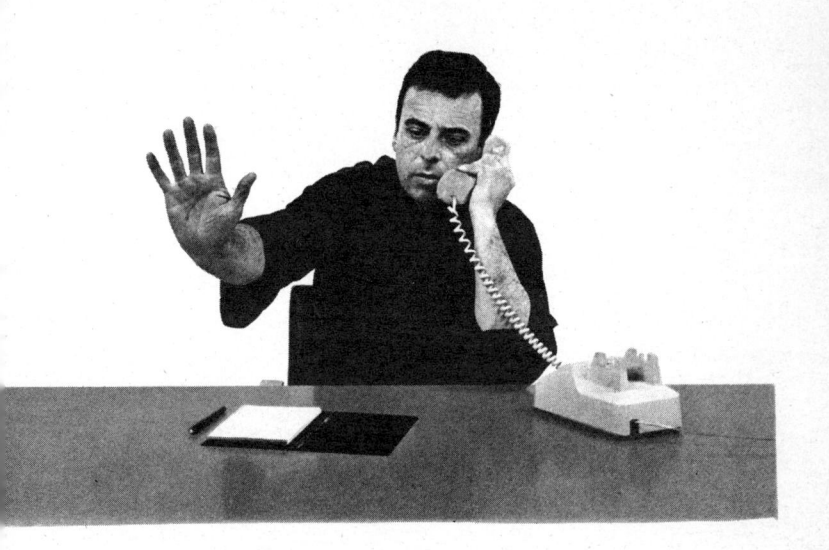

Extend your arm straight out in front of you and place the palm of your hand straight up as though you were going to push something shut. Swing your arm back and forth from the shoulder. Start out with short swings and gradually increase them until they are quite wide. When you begin this exercise, move slowly and then pick up speed. Continue the swinging action for a count of ten.

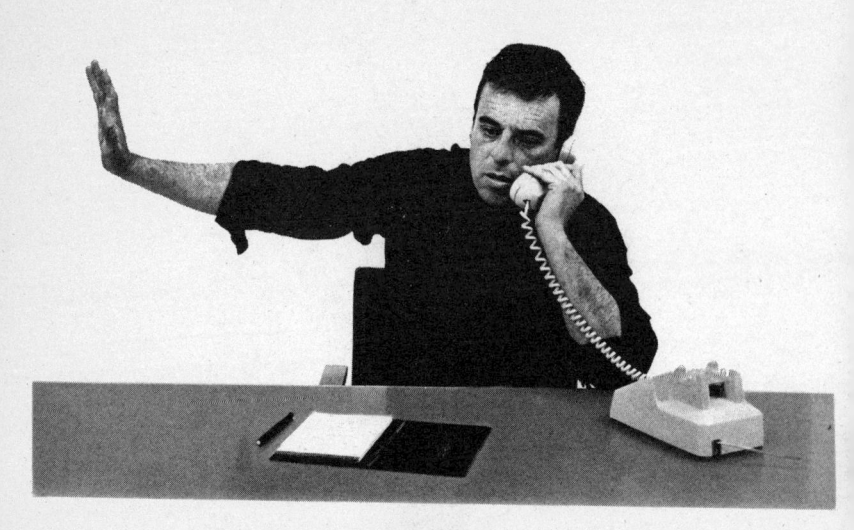

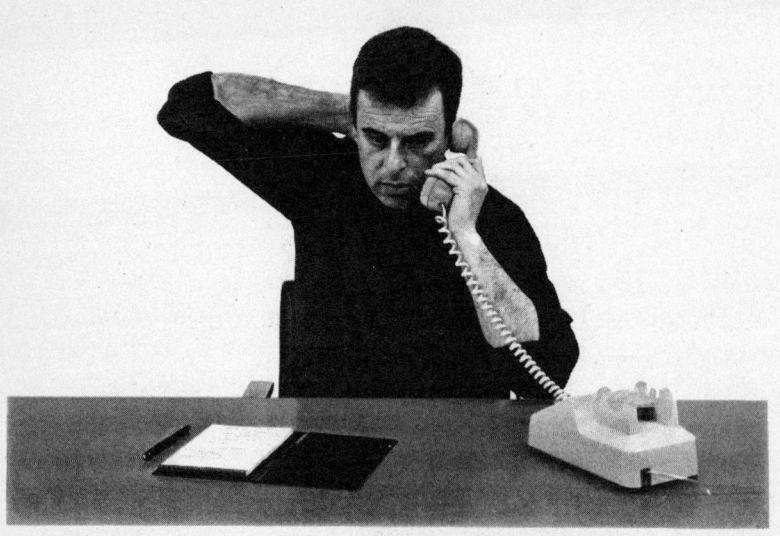

EXECU-CIZE

WHEN THE TELEPHONE RINGS

3.

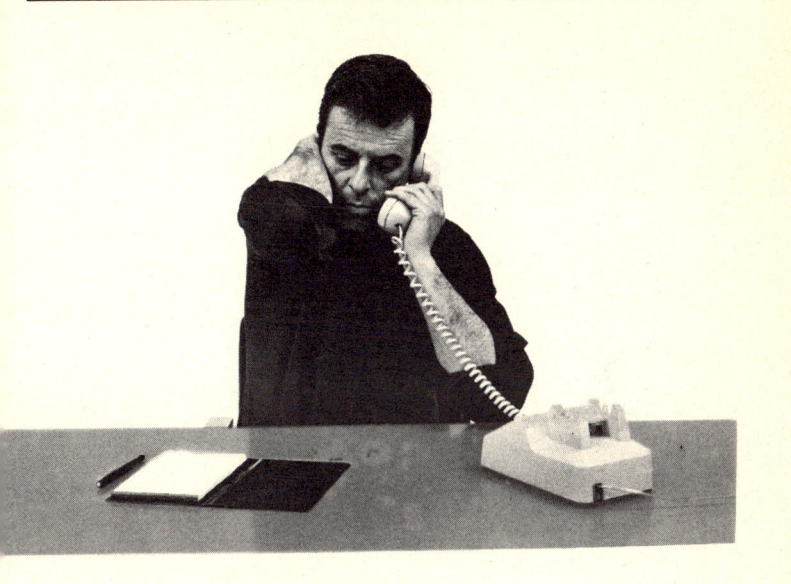

Place the palm of your free hand behind your neck. Use a firm pressure but not excessively so. If you can feel discomfort, there is too much pressure. Ease up. Your elbow should be out straight, perpendicular from your body. Bring your arm in toward your face until it rests on your cheek. Return your arm to the starting position. This exercise should be done at a medium speed for a count of ten.

EXECU-CIZE

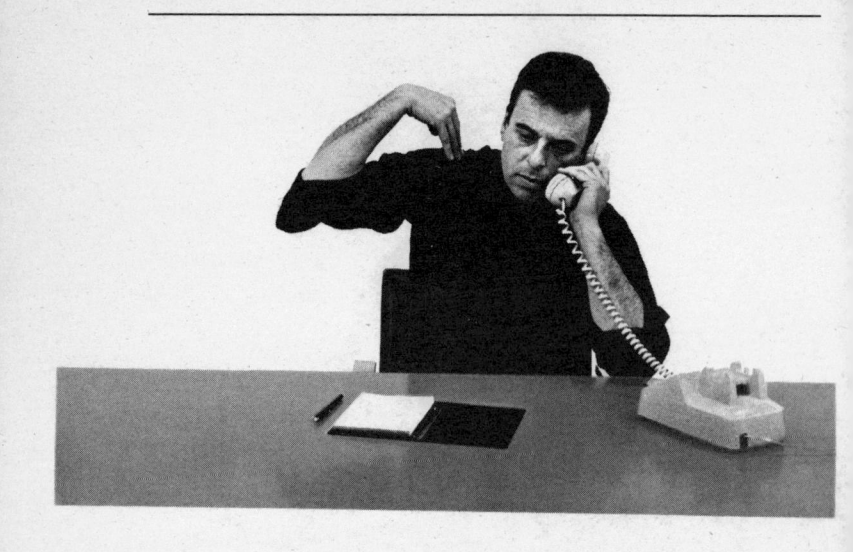

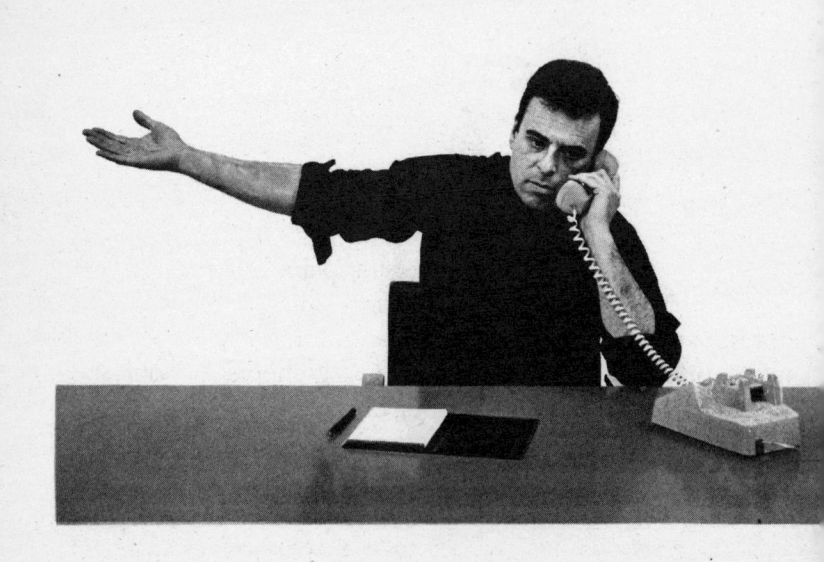

WHEN THE TELEPHONE RINGS

4.

Place the fingertips of your free hand on your shoulder. Extend your arm straight out to your side. Bring your fingertips back to your shoulder. Do this five times. The action is meant to come from your elbow.

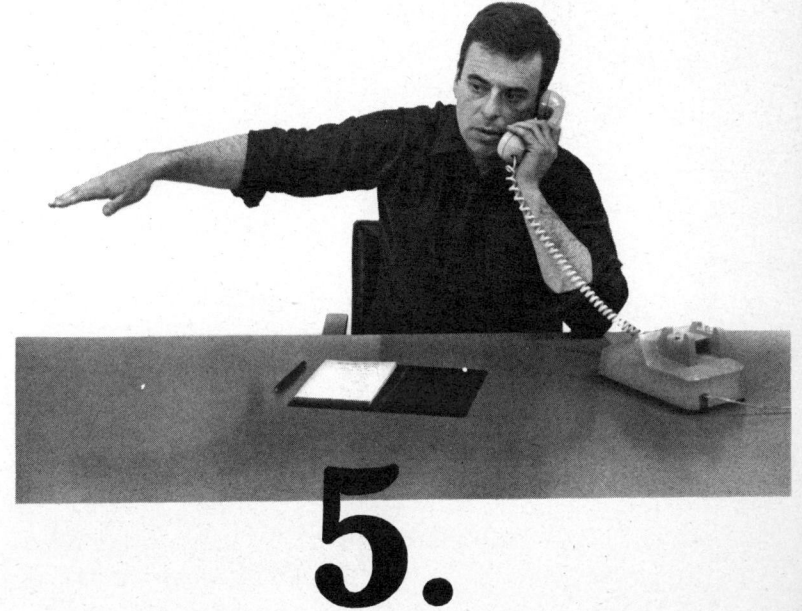

5.

Extend your free arm straight out from your side. Rotate your arm counter clockwise five times and then clockwise five times. The

EXECU-CIZE

faster you can do this action, the better. The motion should, however, come from your shoulder.

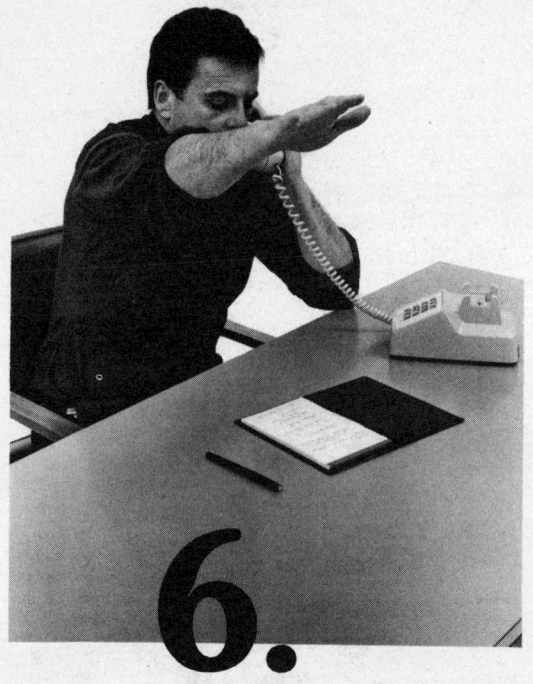

6. Extend your free arm out straight in front of you. Keep your hand open and the palm down. Move your arm up and down as though you were bouncing a ball. Again, this action should come from your shoulder only, and the faster you move your arm up and down, the better. Do this exercise no more than ten times. For a slight variation, spread your fingers open as wide as you can.

WHEN THE TELEPHONE RINGS

7.

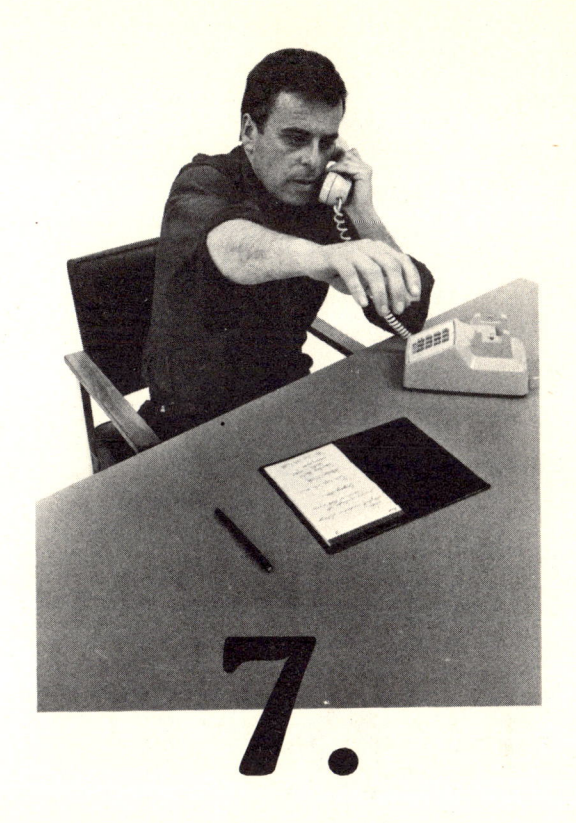

Form your hand into a loose fist. Move your arm back and forth as though you were clipping someone on the jaw. This action should come from the shoulder and the elbow. In this case, your elbow acts as something of a spring action. Five forward thrusts is enough. This exercise also has another advantage for women. The forward thrust of the arms brings the pectoral muscles into play at the same time.

EXECU-CIZE

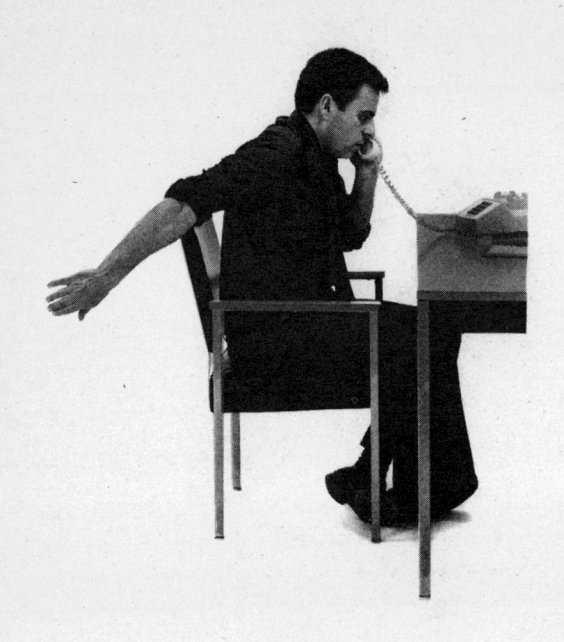

8.

Place your arm at your side so that your hand is pointing toward the floor. Keep your hand open. Tighten the muscles in your arm and swing it back and forth. Start out slowly and gradually pick up speed. Slow down gradually and release the tension of your arm muscles.

WHEN THE TELEPHONE RINGS

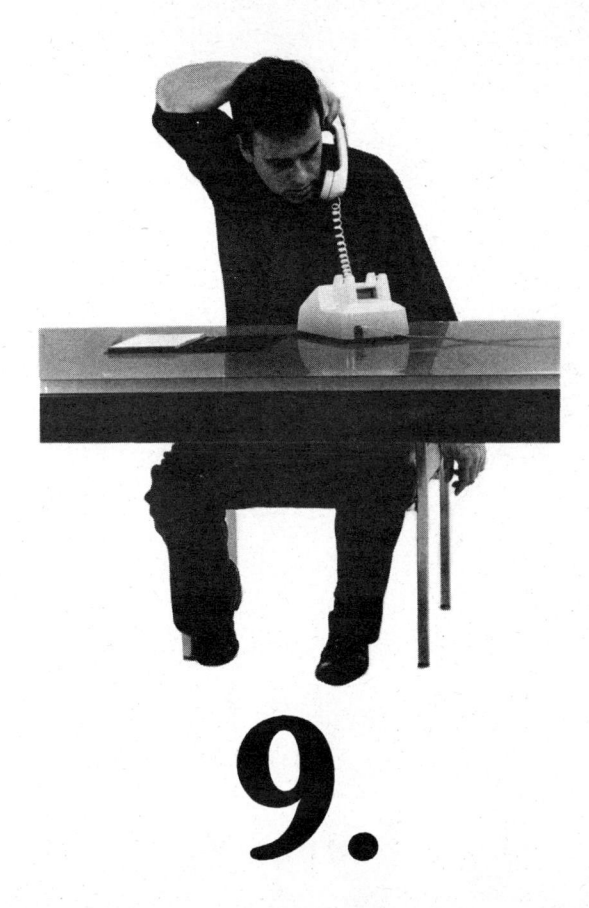

9.

For the sake of illustrating this exercise, let us assume that you are holding the telephone receiver in your left hand. Take your right arm and place it across the top of your head so that you are able to grasp the receiver with your right hand. Release your left hand. Drop your left arm to your side so that

EXECU-CIZE

your hand is pointing toward the floor. Still holding the telephone receiver with your right hand, lean toward your left as far as you can. Your ultimate goal is to be able to touch the floor with your fingertips. Hold this position for a count of five. Return to an upright position in your chair.

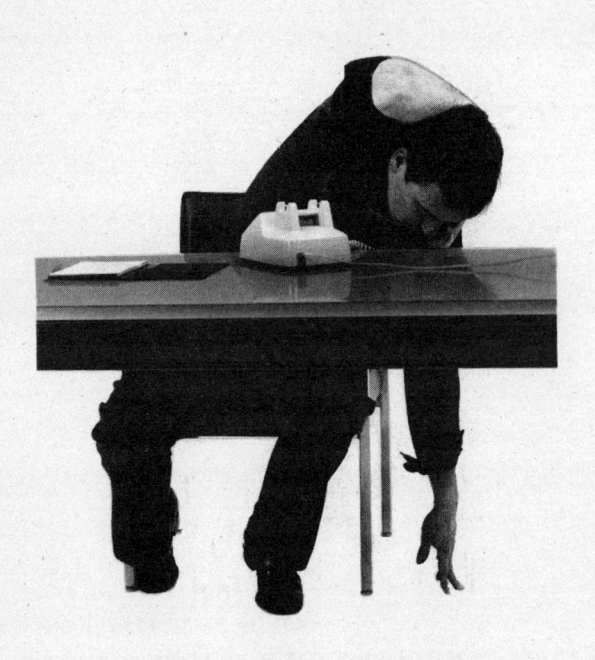

WHEN THE TELEPHONE RINGS

10.

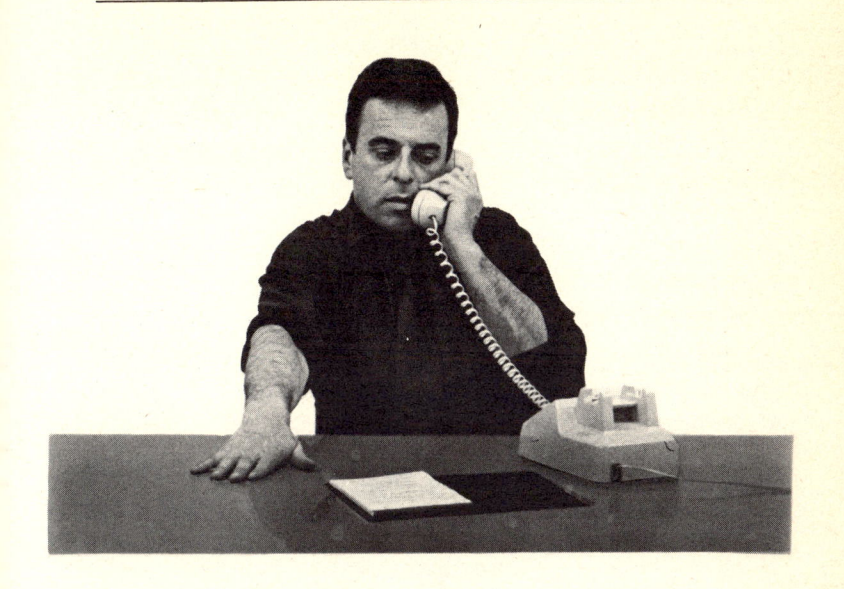

Sit in your desk chair perfectly straight. Take your free arm and reach as far across your desk as you can without bending forward from your waist. As time goes on, your reach will improve somewhat, but unless you have unusually long arms, you will probably never be able to reach all the way across the desk. Trying to do so will only result in pulled muscles.

There are several ways you can do these exercises so that both arms are brought into play each time you

EXECU-CIZE

use the telephone. Let us, for the sake of illustration, assume that you hold the telephone in your left hand. You could do these exercises, one through ten, with your right hand and then switch the phone over and begin exercising your left arm, again doing the exercises one through ten. You can also alternate. Do Exercise One with your right arm, and transfer the phone so that you can do the action with your left arm. Then do Exercise Two with your left arm and switch the telephone receiver over so the action can be done with your right arm. A third method is to use one exercise exclusively for each phone call that you get. For example, during your first call of the day, you would do only Exercise One; you would, of course, alternate your arms. Exercise Two is done while you are handling your second call, and so forth.

If you take or make more than ten calls a day, start the telephone program again, i.e., Exercise One would be used during the eleventh call. Another schedule that you might like is using two exercises each day. For example, on Monday, Exercise One is done in the morning and Exercise Two in the afternoon. On Tuesday, Exercise Three is done in the morning and Exercise Four in the afternoon. All of these schedules, of course, allow you to alternate so that the right side of your body receives as much exercise as your left side. The schedule you choose for these actions does not matter. You should, however, keep your own telephone habits in mind. For those of you who are in and out of the office all day, the last schedule is the most practical because it allows you to make full use of all ten exercises. Those of

WHEN THE TELEPHONE RINGS

you who are constantly on the phone will probably find the first schedule the most enjoyable since it permits variety.

During this discussion of telephone execucizes, I've been talking as though you will *get* all of the calls. Naturally, you are going to have to make a few yourself, even if you just push a button to ask your secretary to put through a call. The automatic tendency, I know all too well, is to reach for the phone set and bring it as close as possible. By doing this, however, you waste an opportunity to really use your muscles. Turn the dialing or button-pushing action into a stretch. Keep the phone far enough away from you so that you have to reach for it. Now, by far enough, I mean so that you can reach to push a button or work the dial easily and yet still keep your arm straight. A straight arm means no bending at the elbow. The straight arm should also be used when you lift up the receiver. Moving your telephone a few inches back from you may seem like a small thing to do, but when you consider the number of times you use the instrument, your arms will get a goodly amount of exercise each day. For the first day or two, this arrangement is annoying, but once you become accustomed to it, having to reach is the most natural thing in the world to do. Each morning, though, you will probably have to check to make sure that your phone is back where it should be. Secretaries and cleaning personnel have a habit of pushing the phone closer to the chair so that it will be more "convenient" for the person who will be using it. It may be convenient, but it is not the way to get yourself back into shape!

CHAPTER 11

EXECUCIZES FOR SPECIAL OCCASIONS

As you have no doubt noticed by now, most of these execucizes are meant to be done in your office while you are alone. I have long felt that having an audience while getting back into shape is not necessary. But as every up-and-coming young executive quickly learns, it is all but impossible to spend every day working at his or her desk alone. There is that unavoidable fact of business life known as the Conference. These meetings can last anywhere from a few minutes to a whole day. Sometimes there is a break for lunch; sometimes there is not. When the chatter continues through the meal, a member of the staff trots in around noontime with an assortment of sandwiches and styrofoam cups filled with coffee. The Conference continues between bites of food. The more enthusiastic conferees don't even bother to break between bites.

EXECUCIZES FOR SPECIAL OCCASIONS

They go right on talking while chewing. What happens to your execucize program during these sessions? Nothing. You continue using a series of motions that are not obvious. Yes, you can go right on execucizing, and no one will ever know what you are doing.

In fact, I find that it is an excellent idea to execucize. These motions keep you alert. The urge to yawn or fiddle in your seat is kept under control. You maintain the appearance of being wide-awake even when you find the whole meeting to be a boring waste of time. And need I point out that the executive who sits in on a conference and yawns hardly makes the best of all possible impressions?

These execucizes can be done in any order. You might, however, want to give special attention to the execucizes that deal with your face and neck because when done properly, they give the impression that you are listening with rapt attention and fascination to what is being said. And you know as well as I do that a speaker loves to feel that the audience is hanging on every word. That is simply human nature.

Here are the facial execucizes that you can use while sitting in on conferences.

EXECU-CIZE

1.

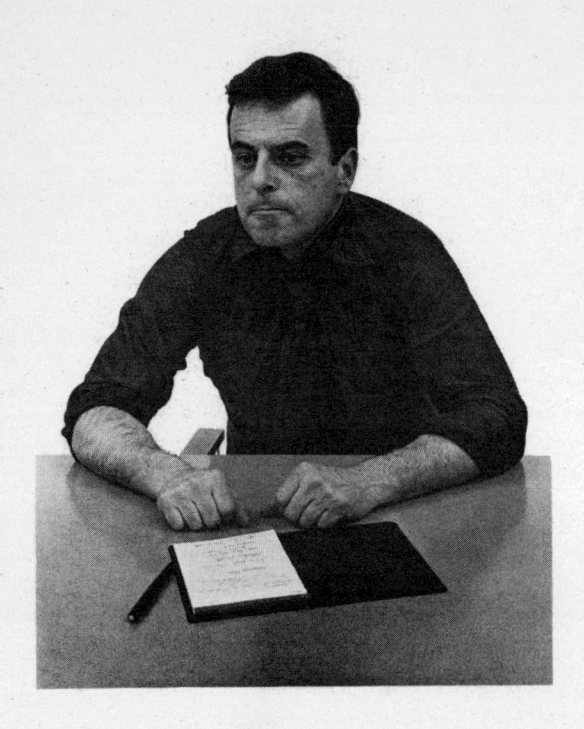

Tighten your lower jaw and gently pull your upper and lower lips into your mouth. Hold this position for a count of ten and release. Not only does this action allow you to firm up the muslces of your jowls, but it is also a great way to stifle a yawn.

EXECUCIZES FOR SPECIAL OCCASIONS

2.

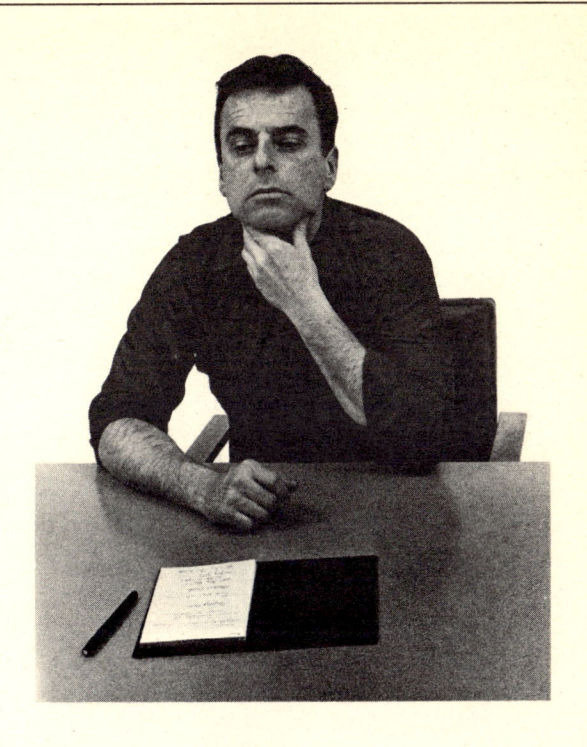

Bend your head back slightly. Tighten the muscles under your chin and hold this position for a count of five. A variation on this is to rub your hand upward along your neck. Place the section between your thumb and index finger just below

EXECU-CIZE

your Adam's apple. Do not press hard against your throat. Gently move your hand up your neck until it is under your chin. Release your hand and repeat the action twice more. This execucize helps to tighten the skin of your neck while leaving the impression that you are giving whatever point the speaker is making very serious consideration.

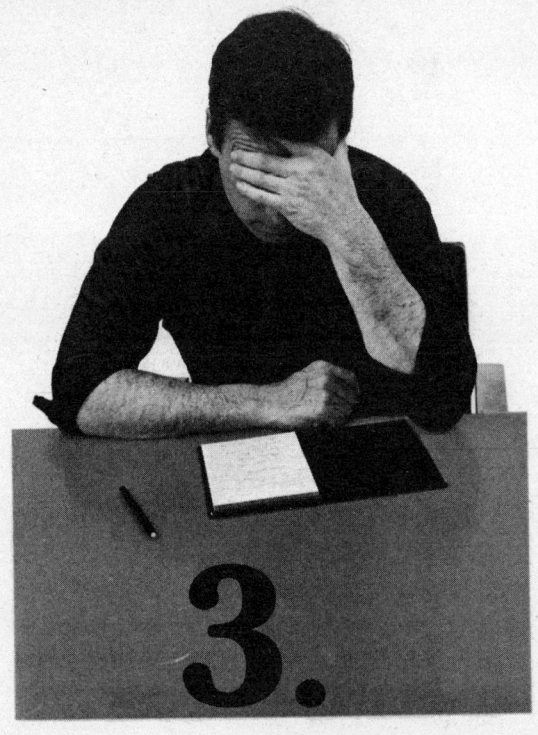

3.

Place your thumb and your index finger just over your eyebrows. Gently tug the skin of your forehead upward. Do this for a count of ten. This

EXECUCIZES FOR SPECIAL OCCASIONS

motion, which is designed to smooth out wrinkles, is especially good when you have been asked to look over some written material since it does give anyone who might be watching the impression that you are deeply engrossed in the papers.

For your arms, there are these execucizes . . .

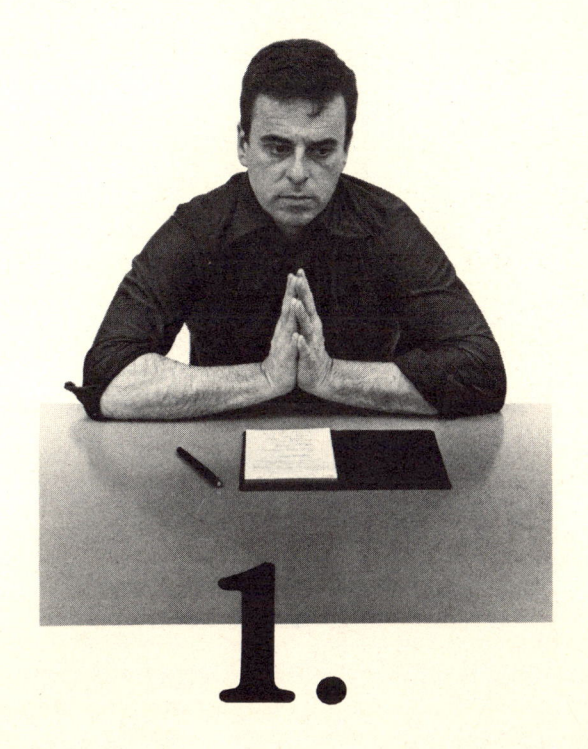

1.

Rest your elbows on the table in front of you or on the arm rests of your chair. Place your hands together and spread your fingers wide

129

EXECU-CIZE

apart. Push one hand against the other as hard as you can. You will feel the muscles of your upper arms tightening. Hold this position for a count of ten and release the tension slowly.

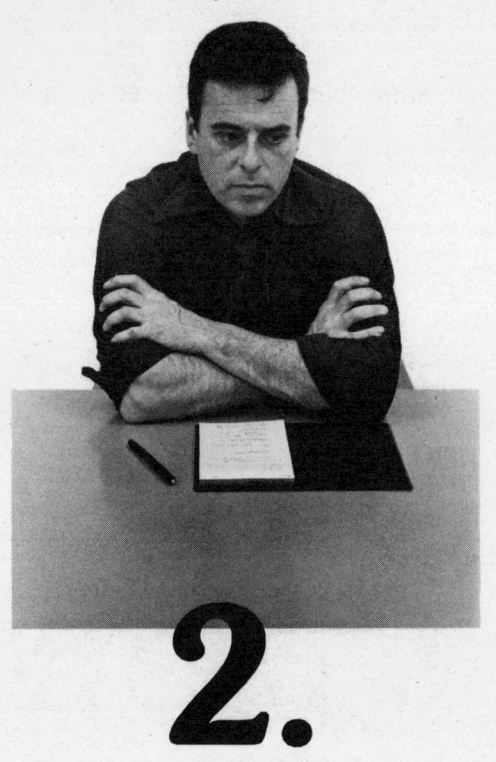

2.

Another type of isometric action for your upper arms is to fold your arms. Rest them on the table before you. With your hands, push against your arms and hold this position for a count of ten. Slowly release the tension.

EXECUCIZES FOR SPECIAL OCCASIONS

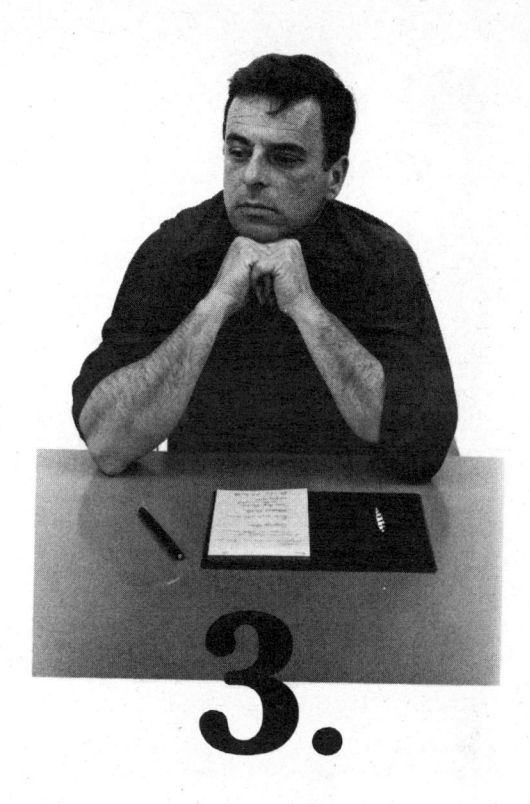

3. Rest your elbows on the table before you. Lace your fingers together so that they are pointing downward. Try to pull your fingers apart for a count of ten. Slowly release the pressure. You can, if you like, rest your chin in the groove that will be formed by your hands in this position.

And you need not ignore your legs during conferences and meetings either. Here are a few actions that you can do while you are in a group around a table.

EXECU-CIZE

1.

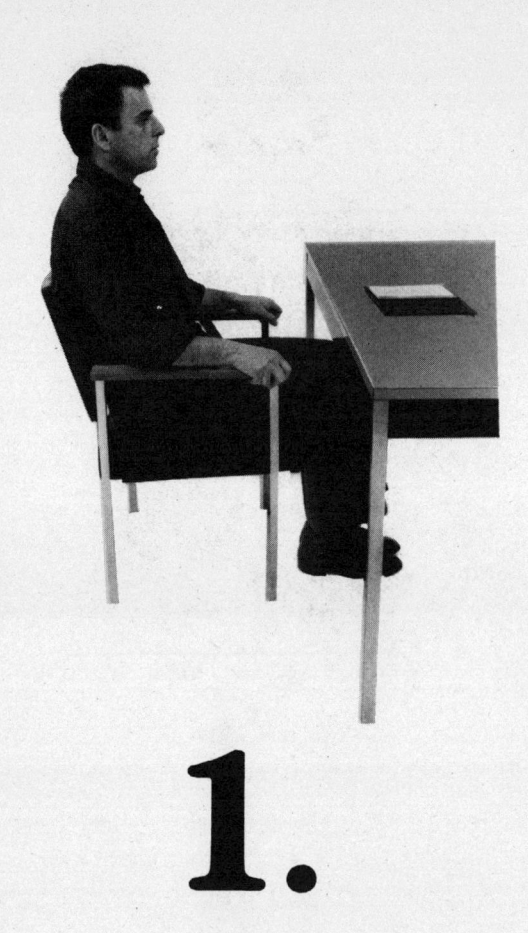

Place your feet flat on the floor. Move them slightly apart. Press against the floor as hard as you can so that the muscles in your calves tighten. Hold this position for a count of five and release the tension.

EXECUCIZES FOR SPECIAL OCCASIONS

2.

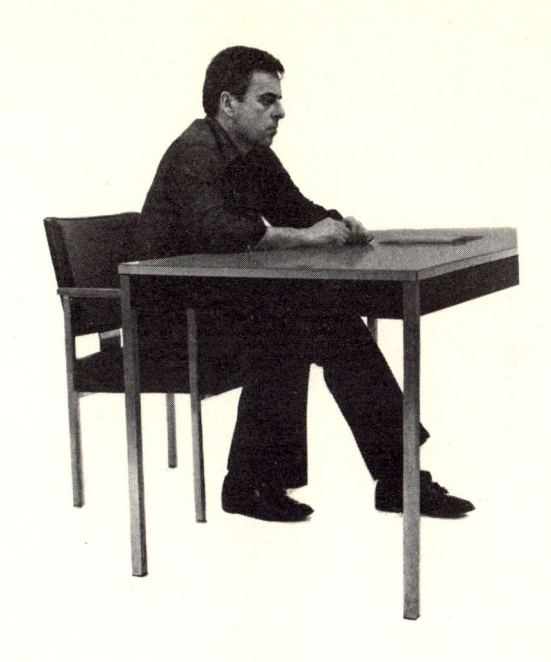

           Raise your right foot about three inches off the floor. Tighten the muscles in the calf. Move the right leg back and forth to a count of five. Release the tension and repeat the action with your left leg. Be careful not to move your leg forward more than two inches.

EXECU-CIZE

3.

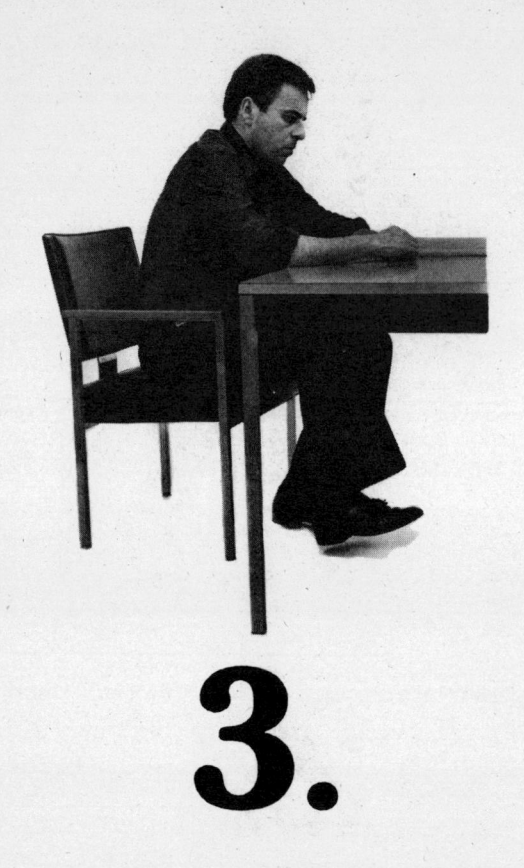

Start out with your feet flat on the floor. Walk them forward for two or three paces. Walk them back. The count is for five times forward and five times back.

And now the final, all-around special occasion execucize. Earlier on in this book, I mentioned that there is nothing like a good stretch to revive your energy and bring nearly all of your muscles into play. Then I went on

EXECUCIZES FOR SPECIAL OCCASIONS

to describe a stretch that required you to stand up. Stretching is also useful while you are sitting in on a conference or a meeting. And while you cannot stand up, you can still avail yourself of this activity. First of all, check to see that you are sitting in your chair properly. Pull your stomach muscles in as far as they will go. Place your feet together and flat on the floor. Lace your fingers together behind your neck. As you push your neck against your laced fingers, also push your feet against the floor so that the muscles in your calves tighten. Hold this position for a count of ten and slowly release the tension. Do this no more than once every hour.

Avail yourself of these special occasion execucizes, and you will accomplish two things—you will help to get your body back into shape, and you will put in your required time at conferences.

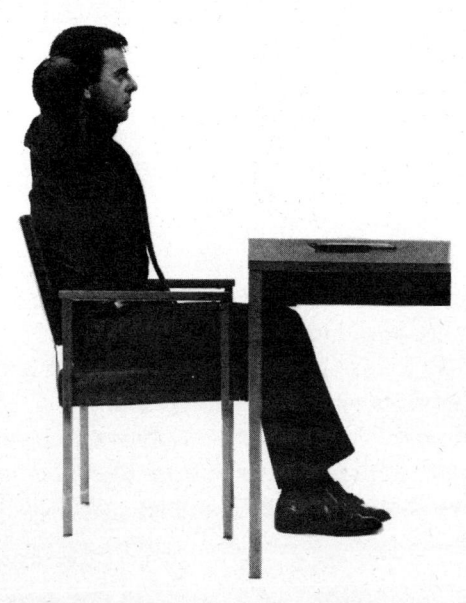

CHAPTER 12

SAMPLE PROGRAMS

These programs cover the three phases necessary to get back into shape. The Beginner's Program is for people who have not exercised on a regular basis for at least a year. Those of you who fit into this category can select either Option #1 or #2. Or you can alternate the two. The first week follow Option #1, the second follow #2. You can also alternate on a daily basis—Monday use Option #1, Tuesday use Option #2, and so forth. Furthermore, your one exercise need not be the same each day unless you wish it to be. The waist action you do on Tuesday can be different from the one you did on Monday. For those of you who like variety, make use of it, Execucize allows it. And if you prefer a set pattern, then establish one. Execucize makes it easy to do that, too. However you make use of the two options available is unimportant. What is important is that you follow the basic outlines as given. That means adhere to the *number* of exercises recommended so that your body is able to adjust gradually to your

SAMPLE PROGRAMS

fitness program. If you are using Execucize to supplement another fitness program, then skip the Beginner's Program and go right to the Advanced Program.

The Advance Program represents the *minimum* amount of exercise that you will need. The more exercise that you do in the course of a day, the better off you will be. As with the Beginner's Program, the options given for the Advanced Program can be varied or not, depending on your preference.

Once you have reached a level of fitness that satisfies you, you have a choice—either continue with the Advanced Program or shift over to the Maintenance Program which is a modified version of the Beginner's Program. Again the chance for variety is made available.

The Beginner's Program: For use during the first two weeks you are on the Execucize Program.
Option #1

1.

Do the stretching exercises described in Chapter 8 twice each weekday—when you come into your office in the morning and when you leave at night.

EXECU-CIZE

*2.

The General Body Action.

*3.

Any one waist exercise once a day.

*4.

Any one waist and leg exercise once a day.

SAMPLE PROGRAMS

*5.

Any one leg exercise once a day.

6.

You may do one telephone exercise (Chapter 10) and one special occasion exercise (Chapter 11) once a day if the opportunity presents itself.

7.

The stress relief exercises (Chapter 9) as necessary.

EXECU-CIZE

Option #2

1.

Do the stretching exercises described in Chapter 8 twice each weekday—when you come into your office in the morning and when you leave at night.

*2.

The General Body Action.

*3.

Any three waist and leg exercises, each once a day.

SAMPLE PROGRAMS

4.

You may do one telephone exercise (Chapter 10) and one special occasion exercise (Chapter 11) once a day if the opportunity presents itself.

5.

The stress relief exercises (Chapter 9) as necessary.

EXECU-CIZE

The Advanced Program: During the third week you are on the Execucize Program, start this program.

Option #1

1.

Do the stretching exercises described in Chapter 8 twice each weekday—when you come into your office in the morning and when you leave at night.

*2.

The General Body Action.

*3.

Any two waist exercises at least once a day.

SAMPLE PROGRAMS

*4.

Any one waist and leg exercise at least once a day.

*5.

Any two leg exercises at least once a day.

6.

At least two telephone exercises (Chapter 10) once a day, and, if the opportunity presents itself, one special occasion exercise (Chapter 11).

EXECU-CIZE

7.

The stress relief exercises (Chapter 9) as necessary.

Option #2

1.

Do the stretching exercises described in Chapter 8 twice each weekday—when you come into your office in the morning and when you leave at night.

＊2.

The General Body Action.

SAMPLE PROGRAMS

*3. Any five waist and leg exercises at least once a day.

4. At least two telephone exercises (Chapter 10) once a day, and, if the opportunity presents itself, one special occasion exercise (Chapter 11).

Option #3

1. Do the stretching exercises described in Chapter 8 twice each weekday—when you

EXECU-CIZE

come into your office in the morning and when you leave at night.

*2.

The General Body Action.

*3.

Any one waist exercise at least once a day.

*4.

Any three waist and leg exercises at least once a day.

SAMPLE PROGRAMS

*5.

Any one leg exercise at least once a day.

6.

At least two telephone exercises (Chapter 10) once a day, and, if the opportunity presents itself, one special occasion exercise (Chapter 11).

7.

The stress relief exercises (Chapter 9) as necessary.

EXECU-CIZE

The Maintenance Program: Revert to The Beginner's Program, either Option 1 or #2, only do the exercises a minimum of twice a day. Be sure to move your body at a fairly rapid speed.

*These exercises are described in Chapter 7.

CHAPTER 13

THE COMPANY CAFETERIA

If there is one place that an executive who is trying to get back into shape should avoid, it is the typical company cafeteria. All the good that you accomplish with the Execucize Program can be undone by eating daily in these places. Notice, though, that I said "typical." Many of the larger corporations maintain specialized dining facilities for their employees. Low-calorie meals that complement a physical fitness program are readily available. A few even offer gourmet feasts. But these are the larger corporations and, therefore, the exceptions. The small and middle-sized companies, if they offer hot meal facilities, have a limited selection that is usually too high in carbohydrates and fats for your purposes.

My own company is a perfect example of this. During one week meat ravioli was served on Monday,

EXECU-CIZE

beef stew over noodles (very little beef but lots of noodles and gravy) on Tuesday, fried chicken and rice on Wednesday, spaghetti on Thursday, and macaroni and cheese on Friday. That is hardly a menu that will help you stay in shape. Of course, the usual assortment of sandwiches was readily available, too. Boloney, liverwurst, boiled ham, and other assorted cold cuts are hardly the stuff of which physical fitness is made. I know a lot of people think these meats are because of the so-called protein to be found in them. Yes, sandwich meat does contain protein—a good deal of it as a matter of fact. But meat such as cold cuts also contains a lot of fat. The fat, as those of you who are with food companies know, is used as a filler. Any nutritional benefits that you may get from the protein is cancelled out by the amount of fat that you will absorb at the same time.

With all the carbohydrate and fat to be found in the average company cafeteria, what are you to do? The safest, and I must admit, the most impractical solution is, of course, to bring your own lunch. When you do this, you have complete control over what you eat. The advantages, though, are usually cancelled out by the disadvantages. "Brown bagging" it is a large pain. You can always go out to eat in a restaurant which offers a wider choice of foods. This allows you to pick items that fit in with your goals. I urge this solution wherever it is practical not only for the choice allowed but also because the change in surroundings, however brief, does you good. It is really not a bad idea to leave the office for an hour or so. Many of you, though, are in a position where "eating in" is almost obligatory. More and more com-

THE COMPANY CAFETERIA

panies are locating in suburban and semi-rural areas. This means getting to a restaurant is quite a drive. And, too, some companies "expect" the executives to use the cafeteria. So when you are "cornered" into using the company dining room, be very selective with the foods.

Over the past several years, we as a nation, have become more fitness and nutrition conscious than ever before. Even the most difficult of company cafeterias now reflects this current interest. Perhaps not as completely as they should, but enough so that you can pick and choose foods for lunch that will supplement your execucize program.

A good rule of thumb for lunch is "Eat Light." There are a number of good reasons for this rule. The more food you shovel into your stomach, the harder your body has to work to process it. And the longer, too. How many times have you felt sleepy and lethargic after eating a big meal? Chances are you will have to answer, "Most everytime." And I wouldn't be surprised. Your physical energies are being channeled toward digesting large amounts of food. The rest of you will just have to wait. The big lunch habit is why so many of my colleagues, and yours, too, are not up to par after lunch. I can think of at least half a dozen people I never call in the afternoon unless it is very, very important. They are all fond of a substantial noon meal. I, as a matter of routine, get in touch with them in the morning. That is when they are running at high gear. By 1:30 in the afternoon, their bodies have dropped into low gear for everything but digestion.

Then, too, all those fats and carbohydrates add

EXECU-CIZE

almost nothing to your general physical well being. You probably take in all you need, and more, at breakfast (especially if your idea of breakfast is a cup of coffee and a donut) and at dinner. Furthermore, your digestive system is probably not working at its most efficient during the noon hour. A good deal of this has to do with your general emotional attitude. The pressures of the morning build up, and you know that you are facing more pressures during the afternoon. If you are prone to indigestion after lunch, the cause is most likely too much food under adverse emotional conditions. (See Chapter 9 for a discussion of stress and tension and how to relax with execucize.)

Noontime is "perfect" for digestive problems. While you are eating breakfast, which is probably not a big meal anyway, you are still fairly relaxed after a night's sleep. You have not yet arrived at your desk to check over the problems that you will have to solve during the working day. And at dinner, the pressures of the day are over. You have a chance to unwind. Lunch is just not the time to make a habit of eating big. Go light. And with a little planning you can probably do so very easily.

As I mentioned, almost everyone in the food service industry knows that people today are more calorie-conscious than they ever were. This allows you to avoid the entree (which tends to be overloaded with useless calories) and the daily selection of dry sandwiches. Check out the salads. Every company cafeteria in which I have eaten in the last five years has offered salads. They make a tasty, light, and refreshing meal particularly if you eschew the commercial dressings which are too oily.

THE COMPANY CAFETERIA

Lemon juice and plain yogurt make good dressings. Most cafeterias have lemon wedges available for the tea drinkers. And speaking of yogurt, a container also makes a nice lunch. Especially today with all the flavors and consistencies that are offered on the market. And, in all honesty, I have yet to eat in any company cafeteria where there was not a selection to be had. Like salad, yogurt has become an accepted and popular food. Usually, though, the secretaries and file clerks buy the yogurt. And ironically, it is the executives who could benefit from it more than they could. Cottage cheese and fruit is a good idea for lunch as well. And don't overlook those little cans of tuna fish and salmon. Again, many cafeterias stock them as a matter of course. A little lemon juice will moisten the fish up very nicely for you. During the cold weather, there is always a bowl of soup. You would be surprised at how well a hot bowl of soup can make you feel on a cold day. This menu can also be varied if you cast a judicious and critical eye over the entrees. Naturally, you should avoid the pasta and stew concoctions so dear to the food service industry and keep a watch out for the acceptable dishes. This way, you will be able to cut down on your calories and vary your foods without going on a formal "diet." Every cafeteria serves foods like meat loaf, hamburger, and grilled fish on occasion. When they appear on the menu, help yourself. Meat loaf should be eaten without any tomato sauce or gravy as should the hamburger. And, too, forget the hamburger bun. Grilled fish is usually done with a pat or two of butter. Scrape this off before you eat the fish. Help yourself to the vegetables,

EXECU-CIZE

especially the green ones. Stay away from the potatoes, which should not be any loss. Commercially prepared spuds usually taste like wallpaper paste anyway.

And, of course, no meal is truly complete without dessert. At least I don't think it is. But dessert does not necessarily have to be from the usual pastry selection of the typical company cafeteria. Indeed, you would be well-advised to shy away from these tacky little tidbits. From a nutritional standpoint, they offer you very little except extra calories in the form of fat and carbohydrate. These are the items you should be cutting back on. From the standpoint of taste, they again offer you very little. Commercial pastries tend to be doughy and chalky tasting. Or so my experience has proven. I have yet to eat the commercial apple pie that tasted like my mother's. Your wisest choice is fruit. Chances are that you need it anyway. If you do not, the extra fruit will not hurt you. As for a beverage, stay with those old standbys—coffee and tea. Carbonated beverages are too high in sugar for your purposes unless, of course, you enjoy diet sodas.

Now with a cautious menu like this, does it mean that you have to avoid going out to lunch? It most certainly does not. On those occasions when you take part in a business lunch—treat yourself, by all means. As an executive myself, I know that these lunches are not an everyday occurence.

For those of you who do not eat in, but who, rather, go out, you will have an even easier time of controlling your intake of fats and carbohydrates during lunch. After all, the whole purpose of going to a restaurant is because

THE COMPANY CAFETERIA

of the wide choice of foods that are available. You know what foods you should be eating. Check the menu carefully and make your selection accordingly. Going out to lunch should not mean, however, a fast-food place. Because they are exactly what the name implies, the menu is limited to those foods that can be kept warm over a longish period of time. Foods such as french fries, clam rolls, pizza. If this is your idea of eating out, you are asking for trouble. You would be far better off if you skipped lunch altogether or confined yourself to a cup of coffee. After all, you can't get much faster than a cup of coffee.

Whenever I give a talk on what I have come to call Executive Dining, I can almost guarantee that I will be asked a question like, "What about my ulcer? The foods you recommend would kill me if I ate them." What about an ulcer? Granted, my suggestions have nothing to do with the gallons of milk and creamed soups and sauces that many people are dousing themselves with to keep their painful ulcer under control. I counter such a question with one of my own. "What makes you think you have an ulcer? Did a physician tell you so and prescribe such a diet for you?" You would be amazed at the number of people who answer, "No," and then sheepishly add that they have a pain in their stomach after eating, and they just assumed that it was caused by an ulcer. Then they go on to explain that their brother-in-law, maiden aunt, or, as in one case, a favorite bartender told them the only thing they could do for an ulcer was to eat bowls of creamed soup and drink gallons of milk.

EXECU-CIZE

Before you put yourself on a high fat dairy diet, find out whether or not you really do have an ulcer. You may not. You may have something else—a gall bladder condition. And if you do, all those dairy fats you are forcing down are doing you a great deal of harm. The gall bladder is an organ that is meant to process all the fats we consume whether they come from dairy products or from fried foods or from meats such as pork. When the gall bladder is diseased, it can no longer process fats as it is meant to. The more fats you shove down your throat, the more pain you are going to have. Rather than risk doing severe damage to yourself through self-medication, take yourself off to your doctor, explain exactly what your symptoms are, and be guided accordingly. And until you check out the situation, stay away from self-medication. If you have chronic indigestion, do not try to find relief in patent remedies until you have seen your physician. Gulping a bi-carb can, under the right circumstances, do a lot of damage, too.

Should it turn out that you do really have an ulcer, your physician will describe a diet that will suit your needs. And it will not be as milky as you think. Should your problem be gall bladder, that, too, can be controlled by a change in your diet; and in extreme cases, by surgery. Even if you should be diagnosed as having "nervous stomach," your physician can evaluate your present diet and advise substitutions and additions. But no matter how it comes out, you will end up eating better than you are right now. Combined with your program of execucize, your new eating habits will help you shed those unwanted and unneeded pounds.

THE COMPANY CAFETERIA

I am also asked frequently, "What if someone notices that I'm eating less than usual, and differently as well? What then? I don't especially want to make a big deal out of a shape-up program." That is, of course, your choice. There is no reason why you should not tell people what you are up to. It is, after all, very "in" to be conscious of your physical well being. I doubt very much, though, that you will be questioned about what you are eating. But if you are asked, and you do want to keep your exercise program quiet, there is no problem involved. Simply tell those who ask, "I got tired of the usual fare and decided to make a change."

Getting back into shape is not difficult at all. Especially when you couple these minor adjustments in your eating habits with the Execucize Program. You can be back in top-notch shape in less time than it took to get out of shape!

CHAPTER 14

HOW LONG WILL ALL THIS TAKE?

This is a question that I am asked frequently. It is a perfectly natural one in some ways. It is also a question that I cannot answer with any degree of accuracy because the really worthwhile things of this world cannot be pinned down to a time limit. Let me give you an example. If someone came into your office tomorrow morning and tried to interest you in a bond issue and finished off the spiel with, "You can double your money in just fourteen days," what would your reaction be? Probably, you would escort the individual right out of your office because no sound bond issue, no matter who the underwriter is, will let you double your money in fourteen days. The same principle holds true for a physical conditioning program. You will not achieve the shape of an Olympic athlete in fourteen days or even in one month.

HOW LONG WILL ALL THIS TAKE?

Getting back into shape is a gradual process. After all, it took you quite a while, probably years, to get out of shape. It was not something that happened overnight. To reverse the situation, you need time and determination. You have to co-operate with yourself and the goals that you have set. Within two to four months, you will notice a definite improvement in the way you look, if you take your Execucize Program seriously. For this program to be effective, it is not a matter of a day here and a day there. And you will achieve nothing if you put restrictions on yourself. Telling yourself, "I'll do execucizes when the sun is shining," or "When there's less work on my desk, I'll get back into shape," earns you a big zero. This is a program for everyday.

One thing that does come quickly is the adjustment or acceptance of the program or whatever you want to call something that is automatic. Once you learn the various actions, adjustment follows immediately. Doing the execucizes becomes an automatic reflex. Execucizing at your desk becomes a habit, and like any deeply entrenched habit, it becomes automatic and unconscious. You do the actions without even realizing that you are doing so.

You will achieve results, in time, as I have and so many others as well. Looking in the mirror every morning or wrapping a tape measure around your waist every morning will not show you a great deal. The process is too gradual. Doing the exercises on a regular basis, however, will accomplish a great deal and before you know it!

CHAPTER 15

EXECUCIZE IN GROUPS

Execucize is primarily a personal program. You select the core exercises and do them as your schedule permits. Except for the first two weeks, you also decide how often you will do the core exercises and how many of the supplemental exercises you use. To follow the program, you do not have to listen to a group leader calling out cheery words like, "Okay, folks! Let's fight flab. One, two, one, two. Bend and up! Up and back!" There is no time limit, and you are not in competition with anyone. Execucize is something you do for yourself.

But however personal Execucize may be, it is not an exclusive program. It can be shared among your colleagues to your mutual benefit. I do not mean, however, that several executives meet together on a daily basis to follow the program. Rather, I mean that you can, if you wish, tell those with whom you work about Execucize. Encourage them to shape-up, too. Let them know about the benefits that accrue to those who are in good

EXECUCIZE IN GROUPS

physical condition. Stress the simplicity of the program.

Having several people within an organization execucizing has a number of advantages:

1.

You are not alone and yet you maintain your independence by personalizing your program.

2.

A sense of group spirit develops that a lot of people like; they are more comfortable in a group setting.

EXECU-CIZE

3.

There is the opportunity for mutual encouragement. Sometimes it is necessary. A feeling of, "Oh, what's the use" creeps in. When several people are execucizing as a group, this is less likely to happen. And should it occur, it can be wiped away by the group quite easily.

4.

The element of time is less important. I mentioned earlier that execucize is not a two-week miracle program. In a group setting there is less concern with time and more with what has been, and what can be, accomplished.

EXECUCIZE IN GROUPS

5.

There is a chance to trade information as to why you are using some execucizes and not others.

On the whole, I've had very good feedback from companies where several executives have started the Execucize Program. If you prefer to know that you are part of a group, this could be your way to achieve it. Talk to your colleagues and encourage them to try Execucize. In time, they may thank you for your efforts.